D0537644

HOME
Allergies

HOME
Allergies
Don't Let Your Home Make You Sick

Property of
DeVry University
630 U.S. Highway One
North Brunswick, NJ 08902

William E. Walsh, M.D.

ADULT AND CHILD ALLERGY PUBLICATIONS, INC.

Copyright 2003 by William E. Walsh. All rights reserved.

Published by Adult and Child Allergy Publications, Inc.
Editor: Betsy Thorp
Copy editor: Pam Price
Cover and interior design and production: Mighty Media

No part of this publication may be reproduced, stored in a retrieval system, or transmitted in any form or by any means, electronic, photocopying, recording, scanning, or otherwise, except as permitted under section 107 or 108 of the 1976 United States Copyright Act, without either the prior written permission of the Publisher, or authorized through payment of the appropriate per-copy fee to the Copyright Clearance Center, 222 Rosewood Drive, Danvers, MA 01923, (978) 750-4744. Requests to the Publisher for permission should be addressed to Adult and Child Allergy Publications, Inc., 1690 University Ave., St. Paul, MN 55104, (651) 645-8182, fax (651) 649-3509.

The information contained in this book is not intended to serve as a replacement for professional medical advice. Any use of the information in this book is at the reader's discretion. The author and publisher specifically disclaim any and all liability arising directly or indirectly from the use or application of any information contained in this book. A health care professional should be consulted regarding your specific situation.

ISBN 0-9631544-1-9
Library of Congress Control Number: 2002094336

As a contractor in the home-building industry over the past twenty years, I have encountered the home defects that Dr. Walsh describes in this book. Many of my clients were fleeing houses that made them sick.

If you are considering buying a previously owned home, you must know how to avoid the homes that make you sick. If you are planning to construct a new home, you must know the correct building techniques that will allow you to live in good health. Proper techniques do not necessarily increase costs, nor does paying a high price guarantee you a healthy home. Only your knowledge will give you the healthy home you seek.

Home Allergies: Don't Let Your Home Make You Sick is not a cookbook for repairing an infected home or building a new home. It is Dr. Walsh's guidebook to the good home, developed from his experiences with patients whose homes make them sick. Read Home Allergies to decide what portions of his advice to incorporate into your remodeling or new construction.

I encourage anyone repairing or building a home to first read this book. I wish Dr. Walsh had written Home Allergies twenty years ago!

Robert Eibensteiner
Founder and President of Kootenia Builders

I enjoyed the opportunity to examine and comment on Home Allergies: Don't Let Your Home Make You Sick. It tells allergic people how a home can make them ill. I met many people who suffered the effects of a defective home when I built the Health House for the American Lung Association of Minnesota in 1998. They came from hundreds of miles away to see how a home should be built; they came because their homes made them sick. If you are living in such a home, you must change it.

Taking medicine or eating correctly does not ensure your health if you suffer from allergies. The best way to gain this health is to live in a home as free as possible of the defects that lead to poor air quality. Only in this home can you and your loved ones avoid the chronic illnesses that change your lifestyle. Only in this home can you enjoy days without discomfort and live the productive life conferred by good health.

If you are building a new home or repairing the defects of your present home, plan your actions carefully. Make sure you prevent the mites and molds that Dr. Walsh describes from reaching out from your walls, ceilings, or floors to afflict you with exhausting illness. In Home Allergies, Dr. Walsh guides you to the information that can improve the quality of the air you breathe and the life that you live.

Mark Biermann
President, Biermann Homes, Inc.

Table of Contents

Acknowledgments

This book and the information it contains would not be possible without the information I gained from treating my patients. I gratefully acknowledge their cooperation. I also thank the family doctors, pediatricians, internists, chiropractors, nurse practitioners, physician assistants, and all the other health care specialists who referred these patients to my care. I appreciate their kindness in giving me the opportunity to meet these patients.

I gratefully acknowledge the professional and caring help of the nurses who work with me now or have worked with me in the past: Arleen, Betty, Caryl, Connie, Corinne, Elaine, Jan, Kristie, Nikki, Peggy, and Shirley. Thanks for your help. Also thanks to Kathy, Deb, and Jill who keep our office running.

I would like to express my gratitude to Robert Eibensteiner, founder and president of Kootenia Homes, and Mark Biermann, founder and president of Biermann Homes.

Both have excellent credentials. Bob is a member of the National Association of Home Builders, the Builders Association of Minnesota, and the Builders Association of the Twin Cities (BATC), where he served as director from 1990–1991. He has been a member of the Minnesota Cold Weather Masonry Task Force since 1986 and has served as a judge for the Twin Cities Parade of Homes[SM] since 1980. He received the 1992 BATC Homebuilders and Associates in Partnership Award, which recognizes ethical builders who exhibit integrity in business dealings with contractors and suppliers. He has won the Reggie Award[SM] eighteen times. (The Reggie Award[SM] recognizes outstanding design, value, and workmanship among houses entered in the Twin Cities Parade of Homes[SM].) He has also been honored by the BATC for most energy-efficient home, best use of innovative materials, and best use of home heating systems in the 1970s energy crisis.

Mark has built Category 1 homes (the most stringent Minnesota energy code standard) since 1997 and is a member of the National Association of Home Builders and the Builders Association of the Twin Cities. BATC has awarded him twenty-three Trillium Awards[SM], which recognize quality achievement in new residential building, two Reggie Awards[SM], and the Reggie Award of Excellence. Most significant for our book, he is the builder of the 1998 American Lung Association of Minnesota Health House®. This house was a cooperative effort by architects, builders, environmental health professionals, indoor air quality specialists, and product manufacturers to design and build a state-of-the-art house that integrates design, construction techniques, and mechanical systems to create a healthier, more energy- and resource-efficient environment. In other words, a modern, efficient, and healthy house for people suffering from allergies.

Bob and Mark are honorable and skilled builders of the type of homes that I would like you to live in. They spent hours reviewing this book and additional hours explaining their suggestions to me. Their comments immeasurably improved the book and I give them my heartfelt thanks.

Finally, a grateful thank you to Pam Price whose extensive knowledge of construction and repair techniques enlighten many passages in this book.

Note About Case Histories

The case histories described in this book are representative of many conversations with patients who suffer illnesses resulting from environmental exposures. They are included to help the reader understand how the home can cause illness and how to correct harmful home conditions. Although the essence of each case history is preserved, the names and certain facts have been changed to prevent recognition of the patients, to protect their privacy, and to better illustrate the ideas presented here.

Sources of Information

Most of the advice that I give you in this book arises from my own personal experiences as a medical doctor specializing in allergy. For over thirty years I have treated the unfortunate people who suffer allergies caused by their homes and the contents of these homes.

Information and suggestions from health care organizations such as the American Academy of Allergy, Asthma & Immunology and The American College of Allergy, Asthma and Immunology were helpful and are included here. At times my suggestions differ somewhat from theirs and when they do, I have tried to indicate this difference by using terms such as "I believe."

The Internet has also been a valuable source of information. Where I feel it may help you, I have included Web pages for you to explore.

Preface

We who suffer the pain and discomfort of allergies desire restoration of our good health and relief from the pain and discomfort of allergies. We want to lose the wheezing that makes everyday chores difficult. We long for an end to the stuffy noses that makes nighttime sleep difficult, relief from the headaches that torment us. We yearn to lose the itchiness of hives or the eczema that makes our skin irritated and dry. We want to stop feeling so tired.

To gain this relief, we must address our special needs. These needs cannot be satisfied by taking vitamins, diet supplements, or herbs; although worthy actions, they will not end our pain and discomfort. The pills, inhalers, and nasal sprays that our doctors prescribe, although they help us, only treat symptoms caused by our exposure to the allergens in the air we breathe and the foods we eat. By themselves, they will not give us the symptom relief we seek. They do not stop the exposures that make us sick.

We can take actions that will fight this sickness. Pointing directly to these actions is a definition of allergy that I use. "Allergic pain and discomfort arise from eating certain foods or drinking certain beverages. They also arise from breathing certain airborne allergens in our homes, workplaces, or schools." This definition points out that foods or environmental exposures cause our allergic illnesses and that to feel well we must find and eliminate these foods and environmental exposures.

How do we do this? I have already told you how to discover and control your food allergy in this book's companion, *Food Allergies: The Complete Guide to Understanding and Relieving Your Food Allergies* (John Wiley & Sons, 2000). To understand food allergy you should read that book, as its instructions will not be repeated here. In this book we will concentrate on learning about the environmental exposures—the various dusts, molds, pollens, and pet dander that you breathe—that cause your symptoms and how you can take steps to create a healthier home environment.

Before going further I should define a few terms I will use. *Allergic reactions* occur when exposure to substances makes us wheeze, stuff up, or itch. The substances that cause these allergic reactions in susceptible people are called *antigens* or *allergens.* Among these antigens or allergens are the *bioaerosols* in the home.

Bioaerosols are the airborne fragments of extremely small living organisms. They include house dust mites (commonly called dust mites or mites), molds, fungi, spores, pollen, bacteria, viruses, amoebas, fragments of plant materials, and pet dander (skin that has been shed). These allergens are tiny; you can only see them with a magnifying glass or microscope. In allergic people, these bioaerosols cause illness such as rashes, hay fever, headaches, asthma, and runny noses. Although the term bioaerosols accurately describe the allergens that we are trying to avoid, it is an unfamiliar word that I will use sparingly.

I will point out actions you can take to eliminate or reduce your exposures to these microscopic particles. If you can reduce or eliminate their impact, you strike directly at the heart of the beast that plagues you: the allergies that make your life miserable. By eliminating these exposures—or reducing them to a level you can tolerate—you will gain that very worthwhile goal: relief of your allergic pain and discomfort.

Do Not Try to Make This Book Your Doctor

I wrote this book to provide you the advice I give my patients about environmental control of their allergic symptoms. I did not write it to tell you how to diagnose or treat your allergies without assistance. Diagnosing and treating illnesses is the responsibility of your medical caregiver. Let her or him help you diagnose and treat your allergic symptoms.

In my practice I try to make sure that each of my patients has a primary medical care professional who has already diagnosed allergy and excluded, as far as possible, any nonallergic illness that may be causing my patient's symptoms. If you were my patient and we questioned the cause of your illness, I would send you to your primary medical care professional for diagnosis. Go to him or her now if there is any question about your diagnosis. If he or she wants help in diagnosis by ordering tests or consultation with other health care professionals, please get these tests or see these other health care professionals.

This Book Features Advice That I Believe Is Important

Many of the topics I will cover are controversial; not all experts agree on their importance or how to manage them if they are a problem. In this book I will not cover all sides of these controversies. Rather, I will give you my own thoughts founded on years of experience treating patients. I will try my best to make the information I present here true and pertinent.

Please understand that my specialty is allergy and not home construction. Due to my lack of construction experience, I may make mistakes in the information I present. I have researched this information to the best of my ability and have asked skilled house contractors to review my suggestions. I believe I have not made significant mistakes. However, as each housing situation is different and some of my advice may not be pertinent to your home, be sure to discuss any questions you may have with a reputable expert in home construction or maintenance.

In this book we will concentrate on the homes situated in the parts of the country that have four seasons: spring, summer, fall, and winter. An allergist is most familiar with home conditions where he or she practices. As my patients live in cold-climate homes, I am most familiar with these homes and the defects that cause my patients' illnesses. I hope that many of the suggestions I give will also help people who live in warmer areas of the country that do not have four distinct seasons.

Before discussing how you can eliminate or reduce your exposure to dust, mold, pollen, animal dander, and other components of harmful bioaerosols, I want to show you why you must try to do so. I can best do this by telling you the stories of some of the patients who have found that their environment caused their allergies.

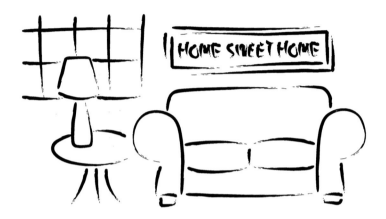

CHAPTER 1

How Your Home
Impacts Your Health

THE FOLLOWING STORIES ABOUT MY PATIENTS will help you understand the supreme importance of the role your environment plays in causing your allergic symptoms.

The Case of the Lakeside Cabin

Jim came to see me at a time when I was just getting my feet on the ground in allergy practice. Even though my fellowship in allergy at Mayo Clinic gave me excellent training in the specialty of allergy, I found that translating this training into practical day-to-day patient care was anything but easy. I was still trying to refine my skills.

Then I met Jim, whose story forever shaped my thoughts and my practice. He taught me the paramount importance of the environment in causing allergic illness and so to this day, I still remember my visit with him vividly.

He came to see me at the request of his doctors, who could not help him. At the age of about 35, Jim was suffering asthma so severe that medication could not stop his wheezing. Only daily treatment with cortisone, a steroid used for uncontrolled asthma, kept him breathing. Whenever his doctor attempted to end the cortisone treatment, Jim's asthma became so unbearable and so threatening that he had to be hospitalized.

Unfortunately, Jim's body showed the ravages of prolonged steroid usage. His face was puffy, his weight excessive, and a lump of accumulated fat sat on his back—the "buffalo hump" that comes from prolonged high steroid use. I'm sure he also suffered the hidden ailments of long-term steroid use: weakened bones and atrophied adrenals.

I confess that I was discouraged. After all, if his doctors—an excellent family practitioner and a well-respected lung specialist—couldn't help him, what I could do for him? With these discouraging thoughts preying on my mind, I started listening to his story and it was quite a story. It was simple and yet shocking.

He told me that his wheezing started five years ago when he spent two weeks at a lake cabin. While there, he experienced a day or two of very mild wheezing. It passed and he felt fine. Four years ago he returned to the cabin and the wheeze returned. Instead of ending after one or two days, it persisted for the two weeks that he spent there. When he left the cabin, the wheeze disappeared and when it left, he stopped worrying.

Unfortunately for Jim, he returned to the cabin the following year. As soon as he entered the cabin, he started to wheeze. Not knowing how serious this wheezing was, he stayed for the whole two-week period instead of fleeing the cabin, wheezing heavily all the while. This time when he returned home the wheezing did not disappear; it continued to the day he visited me, two years later, and it may still be with him to this day.

Jim's history was so clear. Prolonged exposure to the mustiness of a lake cabin brought him irreparable harm. As it was early in my practice I did not know how to help him and I did not help him. Today when I recall Jim's visit, I realize that I should have intensively investigated his home and work area and tried to find musty exposures that kept his asthma going. Limiting these exposures would have provided his best chance to reverse the incapacitating wheezing.

Although at that time I could not help him, I resolved that I would learn how to help future patients like Jim. This resolve eventually led to my understanding of environmental allergies and to this book, with its suggestions on how you can conquer your own environmental allergies.

The Unhealthy School

Jennifer is a 10-year-old girl whose doctor referred her to me because her frequent headaches were so painful that medication could not quiet the pain. I remember Jennifer's mother, and how her face reflected both her grave concern for Jennifer and her frustration because she could not help her. I heard her frustration in the words she used to tell me the story of Jennifer's headaches.

The family had recently moved to Minnesota, where Jennifer was attending the local school. Jennifer's overwhelmingly painful headaches occurred only in the hours she spent at school and continued for one or two hours immediately after she left school; she was free of headaches on the weekends. It was obvious that something at the school caused the headaches, and that the pain would not subside as long as she continued to attend the school.

What made this story even more unusual was that the school had been known to have poor air quality and had been closed and completely reconditioned. It was reopened when tests of its air quality showed that the school air was now healthy. Unfortunately, the school air is not healthy (unfortunately, tests don't catch everything), and Jennifer cannot return to that school.

The Old Moldy House

Wally is a business acquaintance who became a friend. Years ago during a meeting I asked Wally how he was doing. He replied, "Not well, Bill." I know he didn't want to bother me with his medical troubles, but I urged him to tell me his story. What he had to say was simple but troubling.

"Well Bill, I've got asthma, and in spite of all the drugs I am taking, the asthma is steadily getting worse. At first I used cortisone [the same medicine Jim was using] for only a few days here and there. Now I must take it daily. If I try to decrease my dose of cortisone, I can't breathe and must go back to using the cortisone again."

Shades of poor Jim and his cortisone-dependent asthma. When I met Jim years ago, I did not know how to help patients with cortisone-dependent asthma, but now I knew. I asked Wally a question that I had asked Jim, but now the answer meant much more: I asked Wally where he lived.

He told me that he lived in an old house that had a moldy basement. Moreover, not only was the basement moldy, but the walls were moldy. The house had been built before the invention of modern insulation; to preserve the warmth of the home the spaces between the inside and outside walls had been filled with old newspaper and horsehair. I suspected that this old newspaper/hair insulation was moldy and made the whole house moldy.

I told Wally that he had to move from this house and move as quickly as possible. I also told him that he could not expect to improve quickly after he moved. It is my experience that living with high mold exposure causes such a profound asthma that recovery often takes as long as one has lived in the house. For example, if Wally had lived in the house for five years, it could take five years for him to recover.

Because my friendship with Wally continues, I have been able to follow the course of his asthma since he moved from the house. As I expected, his recovery was slow—he improved slowly over the next five years. Now he no longer needs daily cortisone medication to breathe; he uses cortisone only when he suffers a cold that stimulates his asthma. This use is short-term, not like his use before the move— day after day, month after month, and year after year.

Unfortunately, Wally's long-term, high-dosage cortisone treatment left him suffering the side effects of this treatment. Although his facial swelling has disappeared, he suffers from the demineralization and weakening of the bones that results from long-term cortisone usage.

The Indoor Waterfall

Jean is a woman whose family I had treated for a number of years. Jean's symptoms had been mild and she had suffered only these mild allergy symptoms until she took a job as a receptionist.

Jean's workstation sat close to a decorative waterfall. The nearby wall was wet by the waterfall. Mold and algae appeared as a green growth on the wall and were released into the air by the spray from the waterfall. Day after day Jean breathed that mustiness. Day after day her symptoms became progressively worse. Her nose ran, her head hurt, and she felt ill as she answered phones and greeted visitors at her desk near the waterfall.

Jean loves her work and works hard. She did not want to cause trouble but she also did not want to continue to suffer. In trying to improve her work environment, she confided in a friend, telling her about her symptoms and her suspicion that the waterfall was causing these symptoms. Unfortunately, the friend urged Jean to alert the workers' compensation representative of the situation. When she did so, the lawyers entered the picture.

Their first step was to deny that Jean could be sick from the waterfall. They denied that anything grew in the waterfall even though Jean had seen workers turn off the waterfall so they could clean the green growth from the wall behind the waterfall. What a mess!

The Crawl Space

My last story concerns a 45-year-old woman whom I had been treating for three years with allergy injections and medications for headaches. Unfortunately, in spite of all my efforts Jan still suffered daily headaches. Realizing my failure, I sat down with her and we reviewed her home and work environments.

At home, the basement did not extend under the entire house. Her bedroom rested above a dirt crawl space and I believe that the mold from the dirt permeated the bedroom. This mold exposure was part of the cause of the headaches, a cause that we could not control.

Her work area also presented a problem and it was a major problem. Two years ago the first floor of the building where she worked flooded. I suspect that when the flood damage was repaired, the repair was incomplete and much mustiness remained in this area because materials that had become wet and moldy were left in place. Eight weeks prior to my visit with Jan, the roof of the building leaked, flooding her work area and forcing her to move to the first floor. On this floor her headaches increased with a vengeance and caused reflex abdominal distress that became so painful it forced her to leave the first floor and return to the second floor, the floor that had recently flooded. Needless to say, her return to this now musty area did not stop the headaches.

In Jan's case both her home and her work environments contributed to the frequent and painful headaches that she suffered and prevented our treatment from helping her.

What These Stories Mean

These are the stories of five of my patients. They are true and the patients are real although I have changed names and circumstances to protect their privacy. They are not the only patients who suffer exposure to contaminated air. Indeed, most of the patients who come to me for treatment suffer from the effects of air contamination. As their stories show, their homes are not the only source of their illnesses, but they are the only environments they can readily change. Because conditions at school and work are so hard to influence, in this book we will concentrate on what we can change—the home.

For each of these patients, the only way to end their suffering and pain was to correct the environment or flee from it. It may be the same for you. I will either try to teach you how to correct the conditions that make you sick or I will urge you to consider fleeing this exposure. For it is not through medications, herbs, vitamins, or supplements that you will find refuge from your sickness, but only through your efforts to end the exposures that cause your allergic symptoms.

QUESTIONS AND ANSWERS

Before examining the home in detail, I would like to explore some of the questions you may have about home allergies.

How do I know if my home is causing my illness?

The answer is twofold. First, if you suffer allergic illnesses and your home shows any of the many defects we will discuss, it probably is the cause, or one of the causes, of the illnesses you suffer. For a discussion of food-related allergic illnesses see the companion to this book: *Food Allergies: The Complete Guide to Understanding and Relieving Your Food Allergies.*

The second answer is not so obvious until you think about it. If you suffer allergic illnesses, there has to be a cause. *Calling an illness "allergic" always means that some food or environmental exposure causes it; bad luck or the fickle finger of fate do not cause allergy.* If the exposure is from the environment—dust, mold, pollen, or pet dander—you may be encountering this exposure at work or at home. If it originates at work, you will become increasingly miserable as the workweek progresses and feel much better on the weekends or while you are on vacation. If this is not the pattern of your illness, if your symptoms do not vary much from day to day, they most probably are caused by your home (or possibly by both your work and home environments).

I have a rule of thumb that I use to guide me as I try to determine your home's allergy-causing potential: The more pronounced your symptoms, the worse the home allergen exposure. For instance, if your headaches return once or twice a week and are not severely painful, the home exposures are probably only moderately unfavorable. If you suffer daily sinus headaches and weekly migraine headaches, the exposures are worse. If you suffer daily migraine headaches, the exposures are probably very bad.

Similarly, a patient with cortisone-dependant asthma probably lives in a home with severe allergic exposures. A person who wheezes only infrequently, perhaps only with exertion, probably lives in a home with only slight allergic exposures.

🏠 **But I had no symptoms until I lived in my present house for two years. It cannot be the cause of my illness, can it?**

It certainly can be. Many of my patients do not suffer symptoms until they have lived in a house for two or more years. I believe that during this symptom-free time they are slowly becoming sensitive to the allergens found in the house and that their immune systems are slowly weakening under the barrage of bioaerosol generated in the house—weakening to the point that they lose their ability to protect against allergic illness. Unfortunately, a two-year symptom-free period in a new house is not a sign that the house does not cause your allergies. Rather, it is a sign that it probably does.

🏠 **My symptoms have persisted for years and during these years I have lived in three different houses. My present house certainly can't be the cause of my symptoms, can it?**

Yes, it can.

If your symptoms have persisted during your residence in three different houses, it is likely that each house contained allergic exposures that perpetuated these symptoms. Remember, if the cause of your current symptoms is allergy, there has to be a cause in your diet or environment. If your illness arises from neither the diet nor the environment, the cause is not allergy.

🏠 **I told you that my symptoms are caused by food allergy. Why are you so concerned about my environment?**

In many patients, the food allergy that is so apparent in their stories has its origin in the environment. They are suffering from food allergies that would not trouble them if their home, school, or work exposures were not so great that their bucket of allergy overflowed. I will discuss this concept later in the book.

In the next chapter, you'll learn what exists in your home, school, and office that can make you feel so ill. We will examine the allergens that make up the bioaerosols that I mentioned earlier.

🏠 🏠 🏠 🏠 🏠 🏠 🏠 🏠 🏠 🏠 🏠 🏠 🏠 🏠 🏠 🏠 🏠 🏠 🏠 🏠

CHAPTER **2**

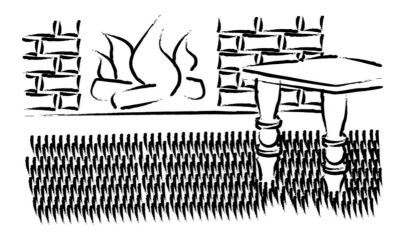

The Causes of Indoor Air Allergies

WHEN WE THINK ABOUT THE BEST HOME FOR YOU as an allergic person, the most important feature to consider is good indoor air quality. Because you spend so much time in your home, the quality of the air you breathe there will progressively promote or degrade your health.

The most important factor affecting the home's air quality is its humidity. Why is humidity so important? Because high humidity feeds the growth of the microorganisms and dust mites—the bioaerosols—that cause so much allergic illness.

Therefore, a home with dry air that prevents the formation and growth of these harmful bioaerosols is the best home for the allergic patient. Will this home with dry air be free of mites, mold, and other organisms? No it won't. No matter how dry the home air, some mites and mold will live in our homes and we will breathe them into our noses and lungs.

Fortunately, even allergic people can tolerate breathing the small amounts of mites and mold found in the dry home. However, as their numbers increase, allergic people lose the ability to tolerate bioaerosols and this loss of tolerance leads to sickness. So it's not the presence of mites and mold in our homes that determines health or illness, it's the amount of mites and mold in the house. That's because the greater the amount of mites and mold, the greater the amount of bioaerosols that will float in a home's air. As the level of bioaerosols increases, our ability to tolerate breathing them decreases. That's what makes us sick.

The above thoughts have introduced you to mites and molds. Now I will look at these cohabitants of our homes in more detail, to let you know what these terms mean. We will start with the dust mite.

Dust Mites

I find the dust mite a difficult topic to think of with comfort, let alone discuss with my patients. That we live with millions of tiny insects in our homes is an uncomfortable and perhaps revolting thought! I am sure that my patients share my discomfort; after all, those who come to my office for treatment take pride in good personal hygiene. They shower or bathe regularly, they wash their hair frequently, they keep their homes neat and tidy. They dread hearing the information that they share their residence with a bunch of creepy little insects.

However, although I don't like to discuss about them—or even think about them—I must. You need to know about these little insects so that you can deal with them effectively. Many studies agree that they are major causes of allergic nasal congestion, asthma, eczema, and other allergic illnesses. In fact, these insects are among the most potent causes of allergic illness.

You may be thinking to yourself, "Dust mites? They can't be in my house. I've never seen any!" If these are your thoughts you are both wrong and right. Wrong because these mites are in your home. Right because you couldn't see them unless you took a sample of the dust in your home and looked at it under a microscope.

Through this microscope you would see tiny creatures that measure about 0.3 millimeters. Mites are so small that three dust mites could dance in the period at the end of this sentence. Their life span is about four months and during that time they lay up to 300 eggs. Under the microscope, you would notice that they are related to ticks and spiders, other insects with eight legs. Their diet consists of the tiny skin scales that we humans and our pets shed every day.

Here's the reason for my—for most people's—discomfort with the topic: It isn't the mite's body that is so allergenic, but rather the fecal matter. Fecal matter that is released into the carpet where we walk, the upholstered chair where we sit, and the mattresses and pillows on the bed where we lie. During its short life span the mite produces about 200 times its weight in fecal matter, a truly prodigious feat.

When freshly laid, the feces are held together by a layer of slime. As the slime gradually dries out the fecal matter also dries and falls apart into very tiny particles. Then, when we walk over the carpet, sit in a stuffed chair, or roll over in our beds at night, these tiny fecal particles fly up into the air where we breathe them. If we have nasal allergies, the fecal particles make our noses stuff up; if we suffer asthma they block our breathing and make us wheeze.

Dust mites are found in every household. Unfortunately, not even thorough and regular house cleaning removes these mites or cleans away their fecal matter. Not even fanatical housecleaning removes them. Mites and their residue are hidden too deeply in carpets, carpet pads, and the stuffing of our chairs, mattresses, and pillows to be reached by vacuum or dust rag. That's why controlling their numbers lies not in cleaning them away, but in discouraging their growth.

By giving you this information, I do not intend to discourage you from cleaning your house. Cleanliness is important for good health. I simply want to tell you that cleanliness alone will not reduce the number of dust mite particles in your home. To reduce them, you must keep the air so dry that you discourage their growth.

Studies show that at a relative humidity level between 40 percent and 50 percent, dust mites die of dehydration in five to eleven days depending on the temperature. At 50 percent or greater relative humidity, they begin to multiply. To completely kill and prevent regrowth of the mite when the relative humidity cannot be kept at less than 50 percent, it must be maintained at 35 percent or lower for at least twenty-two hours of the day if the relative humidity reaches 75 percent to 85 percent for the remaining two hours. If the relative humidity rises above 50 percent for two to eight hours, reducing it far enough below 50 percent for the remainder of the day, so that the house air maintains a mean daily relative humidity below 50 percent, will restrict the growth and allergen production of dust mites.

These figure tell us that to restrict mite growth, we must strive to keep the air in our homes dry.

Mold

Although the word mold is simple, what it represents is complex. It describes a class of microorganisms consisting of a huge number of fungi. Some of the names of molds that you might recognize include *mushrooms, rusts, smuts, puffballs, truffles, morels, molds,* and *yeasts.*

About 70,000 species of fungi have been described; however, some estimates of total numbers suggest that the correct number may be closer to 1,500,000. Truly, this is a huge group, so huge that it forms an independent group of living creatures equal in rank to that of plants and animals. Although their numbers are large and the subject complex, we must try to understand molds because they cause so much allergic illness.

The Molds Around Us

Our exposure to molds, or fungi, is enormous. We react mostly to their spores, egg-like cells that they release into the air to search for a suitable new home. Spores of different mold species fill the air we breathe, both indoors and outside.

The major fungus groups have been divided into over eighty genera. The most commonly identified fungi belong to one of three genera: Ascomycetes, Basidiomycetes, and Deuteromycetes.

Ascomycetes produce their spores in a sac that bursts on contact with moisture, expelling the spores forcefully. High humidity, rainfall, and localized areas of moisture trigger these releases. Yeast is representative of this genus.

Basidiomycetes trigger their spores under more varied conditions and are represented by mushrooms, puffballs, rusts, and smuts.

Deuteromycetes bear their spores on specialized, often recognizable, structures and are represented by common indoor molds such as the Penicillium (the molds that make penicillin), Cladosporium, and Aspergillus species.

Knowing the names or classification is not essential to the purpose of this book, but I mentioned them to help you understand how many molds exist and to let you know how you are exposed to them. Perhaps restating this information will help you better understand this information.

Outside, fungi spores include the large number originating from mushrooms and from decaying plant material. Molds found inside the house originate mainly from conditions that allow humidity to rise. Examples of these conditions, which we will cover in more detail later, include walls wet from roof leaks or basements where humidity is high.

Some fungi are dispersed through water, including the water in rain and the water that spews from vaporizers and humidifiers. Other species live on the surface of our skin or within our bodies. Some live on or inside animals. Molds living inside the dust mite emerge in the feces, augmenting their power to make us ill. Truly, our exposure to mold is high.

Detecting and Measuring Mold

When scientists try to measure the numbers of molds floating in the air of a room or in outside air, they use a technique called culturing, in which they grow the spores of mold on little plates filled with nutrients that molds need to grow. To measure the mold, each prepared plate is exposed to the air and the molds in the air settle onto the plate or are actively sucked or blown onto the plate. There they divide and multiply, forming discrete lumps called colonies, one colony for each mold spore originally in the air. Counting the colonies reveals how many mold spores were in the air that is being measured.

Culturing is not perfect; it underestimates the number of molds in the air because not all molds will grow on these plates. Sometimes it misses so many molds that a moldy house or workplace is declared free of mold. However, we have to use this technique because, if the molds grow in the culture, it does give an estimate of how many molds were floating in the air that we are measuring.

Of all the thousands of molds in the air we breathe, allergists are familiar with only a few. The reason that we are familiar with these molds is that they grow on the culture plates we use and, once grown, can be processed into the skin tests and vaccines used to diagnose and treat mold-sensitive patients.

Allergists buy these tests and vaccines from companies that grow mold cultures in their laboratories. Because the vast majority of molds do not grow on these plates, they cannot be made into skin tests and treatment vaccines. As we cannot test or treat patients with these molds, we have little idea of whether they cause our patients' symptoms and, if they do, what symptoms they cause and if they are major or minor causes. This leaves a huge hole in our knowledge of mold allergy.

This hole is compounded by the tendency of many different types of molds to grow together in any particular home, school, or workplace. Therefore, our questions—Which of these many molds are causing illness? How many molds hide from our detection methods? Do these hidden molds cause illness?—cannot be answered.

In spite of this lack of knowledge, I believe, and most allergists agree, that mold allergy is important. Many studies show that mold-sensitive people breathing air contaminated by high levels of mold suffer increased symptoms including congestion, wheezing, and headaches. The patients that I described earlier all were reacting to mold. To reduce or prevent mold-caused symptoms, high mold levels must be reduced in homes.

Algae

A discussion of molds or fungi would be incomplete without mentioning a member of the plant kingdom that grows in the same places that mold grows: algae. Like molds, algae are microscopic, single-cell microorganisms. It is best to assume that any moist area will contain not only mold, but also algae.

Different from mold, algae are almost never counted during an assessment of air quality. Therefore, even heavy contamination of air with algae can be missed. As they are not counted, their contribution to allergy illness is inadequately studied. Many of my patients show positive immediate and delayed skin tests to algae, convincing me that they are major causes of symptoms and that we need to make our homes unattractive to these guests. The methods we discuss to lower humidity should help to reduce their growth.

Bacteria

Bacteria are another type of microorganism found in home air that can make people sick. They cause human illnesses such as pneumonia, strep throat, and infection of the bloodstream called septicemia. Our focus will not be on these infections; we will pay attention to the allergic symptoms caused by bacteria and their breakdown products floating in the air.

One product, called bacterial endotoxin, is well studied. Endotoxins are the lipopolysaccharide (a molecule made of fat and sugar) components of gram-negative bacterial cell walls. The bacteria release them when they die or when the cell wall is damaged. Sources of airborne endotoxins include many agricultural dusts, aerosols from contaminated water in many industrial plants, contaminated heating and air-conditioning systems, mist-generating humidifiers and evaporative humidification, ice machines, flush toilets, air conditioners, and damp or water-damaged homes. They are common in the indoor environment. Buildings that cause the sick building syndrome often support high levels of endotoxin in the air.

People suddenly exposed to high concentrations of endotoxin can develop fever, cough, and labored breathing. Continued breathing of lesser amounts causes chronic bronchitis and emphysema and makes the airway overly sensitive to allergens and airborne chemicals.

To expand on this thought further, people with asthma suffer the following adverse effects from breathing endotoxins: increased airway inflammation, increased susceptibility to rhinovirus-induced colds, and increased tendency to develop chronic bronchitis and emphysema. This is not a nice contaminant to have in your home, especially if its levels are elevated.

How do we keep bacteria levels low enough so as not to cause our symptoms? Again, we do this by reducing humidity. The measures that I will recommend reduce the numbers of dust mites. They should also reduce the levels of mold and algae, while also reducing bacterial growth and endotoxin production.

Measures to Combat Mold, Yeast, Algae, and Bacteria

I took pains to describe mold for several reasons. First, I mention mold frequently in this book and you should have some knowledge of what I mean when I use this word. When I use it I include all the many microorganisms in the scientific category called mold and I also include the yeast, algae, and bacteria that grow with them. As an allergist I have to treat them all, so I tend to collect them into the single term *mold*.

Second, the more you know about allergies, including mold allergy, the better you can apply this knowledge to your own self-care. Knowing about mold allows you to better understand the allergy these microorganisms cause. It helps you to comprehend the articles about mold that you may read and understand the information on mold that an expert is trying to tell you.

The final reason I told you about the complexity of mold allergy is to let you know why there are no clear-cut measures you can take to lower the mold levels in your home: Some molds will be inhibited if your home is too dry; other might tolerate dryness and thrive; some will be temperature sensitive, others less so. With this many variations, we cannot know all the proper ways to inhibit the growth of these many microorganisms. Therefore, we must simplify our approach to combating them.

For our purposes, we will assume that the growth of most molds will be inhibited by the same actions that lower the number of dust mites. Since the actions that inhibit mite growth are well studied, we can use them as a guide.

You should know about these mold-inhibiting actions because mold causes disease. Many molds and their breakdown products easily float in the air, permeating the air of the house—different from mite particles that are so heavy that they quickly drop out of the air. This means that a moldy basement or shower will contaminate the air throughout the house. Mold allergy must be taken seriously! If someone ever tries to tell you that mold allergy is not important, you now know that you should not believe him.

Mold exposure also differs from mite exposure because much mold can be blown into the house if the outside air is musty. For the mold-sensitive person, closing the windows on windy days when the mold count is high can stop this infiltration.

Cockroaches

Cockroaches have been around for more than 300 million years. While most live in warm, tropical climates, certain species live quite well, thank you, in our homes. Homeowners do not welcome these ugly guests. In addition to not welcoming them, homeowners, especially children living in older buildings in densely populated, urban neighborhoods, suffer asthma symptoms from breathing an allergen in their droppings.

Although high humidity helps cockroaches multiply, they are less sensitive to low humidity, in distinction to dust mites that die in dry air. Therefore, drying out your home will not eliminate them while excess moisture helps them thrive.

The following principle will help you decrease the number of cockroaches in your home: Poor housekeeping helps them flourish; good housekeeping reduces their numbers.

Favorable actions you can take to reduce cockroaches in the home

- Clean your house well and repair defects. Block areas where roaches can enter the home—look for these entries in and around crevices, drains, wall cracks, windows, woodwork or floor gaps, and cellar and outside doors.

- Roaches need a source of water to survive, so replace or seal all leaky faucets and pipes. Remove sources of standing water such as refrigerator drip pans.

- To deny roaches nourishment, keep food in tight-lidded containers and clean and put away pet food dishes after pets finish eating.

- Vacuum and sweep the floor after meals, and frequently take garbage and recyclables out of the house. Use lidded garbage containers in the kitchen.

- Wash dishes immediately after use in hot, soapy water. Clean under stoves, refrigerators, or toasters where loose crumbs can accumulate. Wipe off the stovetop and clean other kitchen surfaces and cupboards regularly.

- Insect elimination measures can be a great help. Ask a trained exterminator to go through the house when your family and pets are gone to eliminate any remaining roaches.

To summarize, good maintenance and housekeeping practices deny roaches entry, food, and water. They will feel less than welcome in a clean, dry house.

Airborne Chemicals

All of us react to smoke from tobacco and wood fires, fumes from cleaning compounds and construction materials, and other airborne chemicals. Some people react mildly, others so severely that the fume exposure dominates their lives. They must avoid clothing stores with fumes arising from fabrics. They must avoid restaurants where people smoke. Some are so sensitive that they cannot leave the sanctuary of their homes. This condition used to be called *Multiple Chemical Sensitivity* or *Environmental Illness*. The American Academy of Allergy, in an attempt to simplify this illness, renamed it *Idiopathic Environmental Intolerance*, replacing a twenty- or twenty-six-letter name with a thirty-four-letter name. Some simplification!

The home ventilation techniques I suggest later in the book will help reduce the concentration of fumes in the home. However, a full discussion of construction materials for the low-fume house is beyond the scope of this book. Please see the resource listing at the back of this book for Web sites containing information about this topic.

Putting This Knowledge to Work

Having discussed the contaminants of the home's air that can lead to poor air quality, let's start examining how you can reduce their impact on your health. We will start by looking at good and poor locations for your home.

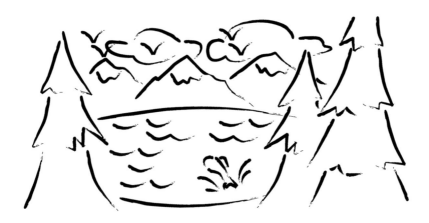

CHAPTER 3

Location, Location, Location: How Home Sites Can Affect Your Health

REAL ESTATE EXPERTS BELIEVE that there are three prime determinants of a home's value: location, location, location. They use this maxim to tell us that where you place a home determines much of its value. An expensive home in a neighborhood of inexpensive homes loses value, while an inexpensive home in a neighborhood of expensive homes gains value.

I appropriate this maxim to tell you that where the home sits is also of primary importance in determining the health or illness of the people who live there. From now on, you should consider location first when you select a home for your family. Whether buying an already built home or building a new home, look at the land on which the home sits or will sit—the home site. Let's look at the factors surrounding where a home is placed and how they can affect your health.

Hills, Valleys, and Sloping Land

A good home site should be on the highest ground you can find. On high ground, a home is continually washed by cleansing winds and the air entering the home is the freshest possible.

Avoid valleys and slopes for a home site. Here the air washing your house may be flowing down from higher ground, picking up the mustiness of the higher ground like a sewer picks up refuse. In valleys, not only will the ventilating wind pick up the mold from higher ground but the air can also be stagnant—the higher ground blocks its movement. Between stagnant air and air carrying mold from higher ground, the air entering your home can be second-rate.

A home site in a valley or on sloping ground subjects the home to another peril: Water flows downhill. When my patients' homes stood in the path of flowing water, it went right into their basements. One patient's home, which had never before sustained water damage, suffered when the landscaping for a new house nearby changed the contour of the land and started to funnel water right into his basement.

Place your home on low-lying land only if all the surrounding land is at the same level so that there is no obstruction to air flow, musty downward air flow, or runoff danger.

Water, Water Everywhere—Lakes and Swamps

Who can resist living on a beautiful lakeshore? Or pass up the chance to buy a really nice but low-priced home near a pond or swamp, especially if the swampland has been reclaimed and the home site looks like a park? You may be tempted to place your home there.

Don't do it. These sites are not good for you. If you buy a home near a pond, lake, or swamp—or on land reclaimed from a swamp—the water table is likely to be high, perhaps close to the slab of your home. If so, this water will seep up into the slab, bringing to your home mustiness with its attendant mites and mold. Even if the water table is low, the humidity arising from the nearby pond, lake, swamp, or reclaimed swamp will probably moisten the air surrounding your home, bringing musty air into your home.

The Water Table

I have already mentioned the water table. However, it is so important that I want to explore it further. The water table is the level to which water rises in the ground. (Capillary action draws water from the water table to wet the ground for a few centimeters above the water table.) Below the water table the ground is saturated with water, above it the ground is dryer.

You should always try to determine where the water table rests and place your home well above it. To determine where the water table lies on a site you are considering, hire a soil testing firm (check with your builder, the local builders association, or the phone book for firms in your area).

The lower the water table the better, preferably well below the house footings and the basement slab. During rains, the water table can rise and, if it is just below the house, the rising water can wet the footings and slab. Wet footings and slab will conduct significant moisture into your home, encouraging mite and mold growth.

Woods, Forest, and Trees

Selecting a home site in the woods or in a forest shows your appreciation for nature's beauty, but not your wisdom. Woods or forests are musty; the winds bathing the forest wash the home with this mustiness. Closely spaced trees block the movement of air, impeding the wind-born ventilation so necessary for the dry house.

If the home must be in woods or forest, thin bushes and trees to allow air flow to the house. From the trees that remain, remove the bottom branches to allow for freer movement of air.

The Landscape

You will waste all your efforts to place your home on a favorable plot of ground if you do not provide good landscape drainage. How the ground slopes away from the house will determine if rain and snow-melt drain away from the house or settle around it and pool under the basement floor. The ground should slope away from the home on all sides to shed water running from the roof. A home site that is on flat ground or in a depression cannot shed this water. Water will probably pool around the foundation of the home and leak into the basement, turning not only the basement but the entire house musty—and bringing the allergic patient much illness.

To assure that the water flows away from the house, install and maintain well-functioning gutters, downspouts, and downspout extensions. Absent or poorly functioning gutters, downspouts, and extensions do not channel water to where it can drain away from that house and are defects that must be repaired as soon as they are discovered. Be sure to examine the functioning of all of these components during a heavy rain to ensure that water truly flows away from your home. If you need to be outside to make this observation, do so only when lightning is not present.

Gutters have several drawbacks. If they are not carefully watched, they can become plugged up with leaves and other debris. Be sure to keep them clean. If they are hard or dangerous to access, consider installing a cover that allows rain and snowmelt to pass into the gutter while preventing leaves from entering. In addition, gutters often contribute to the ice dams that form on the roof in winter.

If you decide not to install gutters and downspouts, but to rely on landscaping to carry water away from the house, be very careful of how you design this landscaping. Around the house, you must slope the ground away from the house for ten feet. The soil should drop one inch per half-foot over the first four feet, then drop one inch per foot over the next six feet. Driveways, walkways, and patios should also slope away from the house, dropping one inch over every four feet.

To develop this slope, first try to determine if construction materials or other trash has been dumped into the space around the basement before the space was filled with dirt. If so, remove it. Then bring in dirt to fill any depression and to create the slope, packing the dirt tightly. If you wish to place mulch around the foundation, first lay down landscape fabric to keep the mulch from sinking into the soil. If the new soil around the house does settle, remove the mulch and landscape fabric before you regrade. If you just place more mulch over the old, water will find its way under the new mulch, flow toward the house, and into the basement. It happened to one of my patients. (See chapter 9, "The Roof and Walls of the House," for more information about drainage around the house.)

Now that we have looked at your home's location, let's explore how your home sits on that land and how that can affect your indoor air quality.

Factors to Consider When Selecting a Home Site

Site Feature	👍 Look for...	👎 Avoid...
Hills, valleys, and slopes	...a site in an open and preferably high location that is cleansed by the wind.	...a site where airflow to the home is obstructed by higher ground or where the slope of the land directs water or musty air to the home.
Water features	...a site far away from ponds, swamps, and lakes.	...nearby water that may wet your slab or expose you to musty air.
Water table	...a site where the water table is at least one foot below the footings.	...a site where the water table is high enough to moisten the footings and slab.
Trees	...a site without trees or with well-spaced shade trees.	...heavily wooded or forested home sites.
Gutters	...properly installed and maintained gutters.	...inefficient, malfunctioning, or absent gutters.
Landscaping	...a site with proper grading to disperse water away from the foundation.	...landscaping that channels water toward the foundation.

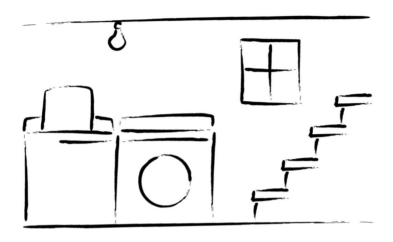

CHAPTER 4

The Basement: Potential for Great Trouble

IT WAS 1925 AND DR. IMA SCHTINKER HAD A PROBLEM. He had a distinct lack of patients. The walls of his office held his certification from The Board of Allergy and his diploma from The Medical School of the University of Southern Florida at Upper Ipswitch, but these walls looked down on an empty examining room.

Not possessing good insight, he did not attribute the empty room to patients' distrust of the legitimacy of his diplomas (they weren't legitimate) or to the odiousness of his personality (it was odious). Instead, he decided that too few people suffered from allergy and he decided to change that. If he could persuade people to live on the concrete slab of their houses, they would become allergic and plenty of patients would fill his empty room.

Unfortunately for Ima, the people of 1925 never fell for his ploy. They remembered the dirt-floored shanties that they or their parents grew up in and the illnesses caused by these dirt floors. They knew that concrete is just pretty dirt and that this pretty dirt belonged in the basement, not under their living room carpet.

Poor Ima, his devious plan never worked during his hapless medical career but it is working today. Unfortunate patients now pour into allergists' offices, suffering the illnesses that afflict people who live on the concrete slabs of their houses.

The above story is factitious and facetious but it does serve to introduce the problems of the basement. As the basement is the foundation of the home, it is also the foundation for allergic health or illness. I cannot overemphasize the basement's great impact on your health. If your basement is musty, your home is musty and you will suffer congestion, wheezing, headaches, and any of the other afflictions that plague the allergy sufferer.

These thoughts can be taken further by asking a question. Can a non-allergic person spend years in a home with a musty basement without reacting to this mold? In other words, will a non-allergic person become allergic in a home with a musty basement? I have seen this happen too often to doubt that the answer is yes. Moldy houses make people allergic. It happens so often that I believe that the non-allergic person living above or in a musty basement is, in that old cliché, an accident waiting to happen.

Please recognize one caution that is commonly misunderstood: *Even if you seldom go into your basement, you can still suffer from its humidity, mites, and mold. It is true that your suffering will be less if you avoid being in the basement; however, it is still a great disadvantage to live above a musty basement—basement air circulates through the house.*

If a musty basement makes a non-allergic person allergic, what must it do to the allergic person? Unfortunately, the answer is that it makes his symptoms so much worse. To help you avoid this suffering, I will point out favorable and unfavorable aspects of a basement.

In addition to examining the basement, we need to take a look at the furnace and air conditioner, as well as the humidifier, air exchanger, and air cleaner that use the same ducts to circulate air throughout the house. They are important because the air they circulate includes air from the basement. They are so important that I will discuss these air-handling appliances in the next chapter. For now, let's focus on the basement itself.

The Case Against Slab Construction

The concrete that forms a basement continually transmits moisture from the surrounding ground into the home in the form of humidity. This humidity nourishes the mites and mold that cause allergic symptoms. Speaking solely as an allergist, I believe the reason your house has a basement is to separate your living areas on the first and second floors from this concrete. It is a barrier to the flow of humidity from the slab to all the home accoutrements on the upper floors that this humidity otherwise would make musty—carpets, upholstered furniture, bedding materials, and other items that can harbor mites and mold.

If a home has no basement or crawl space, the living area is directly on the slab and subject to the humidity passing through the slab. Take extra care in constructing this house.

In the house without a basement, the concrete slab on which the house rests should rise at least eight inches above the final grade of the yard. Grade the yard to drain rain and snowmelt away from the house. Install a tough polyethylene vapor barrier (minimum thickness of 6 mil) under the slab and take special care to seal the vapor barrier to all floor penetrations. Below this vapor barrier should be a layer of fill called ¾-inch minus (that means each piece is ¾ inches in diameter or smaller). This fill will help keep the water table below the slab and it assures a good drainage system to carry away water that may pool below the slab. Perhaps most important, it provides a capillary break. That is, by isolating the slab from the soil, it inhibits the slab from soaking up ground moisture.

Even with these precautions, a slab should be regarded with suspicion. Some error in construction may allow humidity to pass through the slab. Cover it with tile, not wall-to-wall carpet and pad as they become musty from humidity if the slab is not totally isolated from ground moisture.

The Well-Constructed Basement

Laying a vapor barrier before pouring the slab is a good idea and advocated by experts in home construction. The barrier will resist the movement of moisture into the slab and lessen the humidity released into the basement by the slab. Alternatively, some builders lay rigid foam insulation before pouring the slab.

I also believe that waterproofing and insulating the basement walls on the outside is a good idea. One waterproofing product that one of my contractor-reviewers mentioned favorably is Poly-Wall, as it stands up well to the abuse that can happen when insulating and backfilling the basement walls. Rigid foam insulation is then often applied over the waterproofing material. Insulation designed for the outside of basement walls is often grooved to help route water down to the footing drain. A well-designed footing drain is essential to carry away the water that wants to rest against slab, footings, and insulation. All of these products—the waterproofing, insulation, and footing drain—act together to prevent ground moisture from seeping into and through the foundation walls and slab.

You would be wrong to allow the external vapor barrier and insulation to lead you to disregard the precautions I describe. The moisture barrier is only a partial barrier, slowing but not stopping the flow of moisture into the slab and the basement walls. Further, it may have been damaged in installation or after it was installed. With the passage of time, settling of the house or the actions of soil chemicals, insects, and burrowing animals may destroy its integrity.

I want to discuss this idea further. Even with a moisture barrier, whether protecting a full basement or a slab resting on the ground, expect some extra humidity to arise from the basement slab. Some mites and mold may grow in walls, ceilings, carpets, upholstered furniture, and other objects in the area over the slab. If you installed moldable objects in these areas and they did not become moldy in the first year, they could become moldy in the years that follow.

Further, barriers will not protect your basement from flooding caused by a failed sump pump or a broken pipe. This catastrophe will wet and turn moldy all the treasures you placed in the basement. If they become wet from this water, you must remove them from the basement and discard them, losing all the money you invested in them. Once wet, you can never be sure that, when dried, they are not full of mold.

If your basement is bare, if you have avoided adding interior walls to the basement, installing ceilings, laying carpets, or importing upholstered furniture and other moldable objects, you just wipe up the water and walk away. The moral of the story is this: Consider all other options before placing these objects there in the first place.

Note: You can protect the house from water entering through a window well. Install a drainpipe in the window well under a layer of rock and connect the drainpipe with the drainage system you installed at the basement footings. Water entering the window well will drain away through the drain tile. Install a removable barrier (never do anything to reduce the opening size of an egress window) at the base of the window to prevent excess water from pouring over the bottom of the window into the basement.

The Four-Level Home and Homes with Tuck-Under Garages

As an allergist, I dread these home designs. Bringing a garage into your basement, as happens in the house with a tuck-under garage, subjects your home to all of the mustiness and fumes of the garage. An attached garage, separated from the house by an intact wall, does not expose the home to the same possibility of fumes and mustiness entering the home from the garage. Do not buy a home with a garage in the basement even if the home is separated from the garage by a fume/humidity barrier. How perfect is the barrier? How long will it last? Do not place yourself in the position to discover the answers to these questions.

I also fear the four-level home with two levels on concrete slabs. Both of these levels are basements. (Again, speaking as an allergist, not a builder, I consider any area of a house with a concrete floor in contact with the ground a basement). Instead of one basement, the house has two. Unfortunately, homeowners tend to treat only the lowest level as a basement. They convert the higher level into living space with carpets, upholstered furniture, closets and clothes, bedding materials, and all the other objects that shouldn't be in basements. Avoid these houses.

Wood Foundations

Too few of my patients live in a house with a wood foundation for me to know if wood is better or worse than concrete. However, I worry about the ability of a wood foundation to resist mold growth. If it does, how long will it resist this growth? Ten years? Twenty years? Fifty years? Always? What about the chemicals used to treat the wood, will they expose the homeowner to harm? Will some peculiar illness arise in people living in homes with wood foundations? Will animals gnaw through the wood walls? I cannot answer these questions. Until they are answered, I believe that the concrete foundation is best.

Crawl Spaces

For me, crawl spaces are an invention of the goblin that causes allergy. Crawl spaces should not be in the homes of allergic people.

In many homes, adequate inspection, ventilation, and dehumidification of crawl spaces is difficult and in others almost impossible. The humidity and mold in crawl spaces can penetrate the home and permeate its air.

If the ground is wet, gallons of water a day—in the form of humidity—can be released into a home with an exposed-earth crawl space or basement floor. Even if they are covered with rock, they can release substantial quantities of moisture. Earth floors should therefore always be covered with polyethylene and rock or, even better, concrete. Seal the concrete to further reduce the amount of humidity passing through the floor into the home.

Building codes may specify that crawl spaces be vented to the outside. If your crawl space is, make sure that crawl space vents work and are not blocked. If your air conditioning ductwork runs through the crawl space, consider closing the crawl space vents during the summer when the air conditioner is active. Alternatively, you can insulate the ducts. Either measure will help reduce condensation that adds to the moisture problem. Using vent fans in crawl spaces during the summer when humidity is high may draw this excess humidity into the crawl space and from there into the rest of the home. Use fans only when outside humidity is well below 50 percent. Mechanical dehumidifiers reduce humidity in basements, but they are useless in crawl spaces when vents are open.

If crawl spaces are not vented to the outside, I believe they must be vented into the house. I do not believe they can be simply closed off and forgotten. When venting to the inside, moisture- and humidity-proof the crawl space as perfectly as possible and keep air moving freely through it.

To avoid all these problems, I recommend you avoid living in homes with crawl spaces.

A Heating System Installed in the Slab

If you want to heat the slab, use only enclosed systems such as plastic tubing filled with water. Do not install forced air heat ducts in the slab as they are difficult to install and can become filled with mold. If so, as my patients have discovered, they have to be plugged with concrete and a different heating system utilized.

Coverings for the Basement Floor

Many options exist for covering a basement floor, including wood flooring, paint, tile, or resilient flooring (linoleum or vinyl). I believe that installing a wood floor over the slab is a mistake. It hides any mold forming on the slab, and is susceptible to rot. Hygroscopic (water attracting) materials—such as wood—absorb moisture from the slab. This humidity absorption will occur even in winter in a wood floor above a concrete slab. These materials also absorb increasing amounts of moisture from the air as the relative humidity increases. In regions with elevated summer and fall humidity, a wood floor can absorb an additional 4 to 5 percent of its weight in moisture, helping mold grow.

Applying a moisture-retarding paint or concrete sealer to the basement floor is acceptable. I believe that linoleum and vinyl are unacceptable coverings for the basement floor, as they can become moldy. Tiles are acceptable, but the homeowner should be prepared for that inevitable day when the basement floods. Plastic tiles are a poor choice as the water can lift them. Ceramic tiles are cemented to the floor and become part of it, and are therefore exceedingly resistant to separating from the floor with flooding. This tight bonding also prevents mold from growing under the ceramic tile.

Basement Foundation Walls

I firmly believe that foundation walls, the concrete or masonry block walls that the house rests on, should not have their inside surfaces covered. Although insulating and covering these walls helps retain heat in cold climates and improves the appearance of the basement, the insulation and drywall can become musty and permit undetected water leakage. If the wall is not covered, the cover cannot hide leakage and become moldy. The uncovered basement wall allows the homeowner to easily spot any leakage of water into the basement; once identified, the conditions causing the leak can be corrected.

Be aware that bare basement walls are cooled from the surrounding ground. In warm weather, moisture will condense on these walls, breeding mold. Be sure that you continuously operate your dehumidifier in warm weather to retard this moisture condensation. We will further discuss dehumidifiers later.

Partition Walls and Ceilings in a Basement

One of the most tragic mistakes many of my patients have made is to "finish" their basements. This is especially so in older houses. Finishing means covering the concrete or block walls by installing studs, insulation, and a vapor barrier, then covering that with drywall or paneling. Interior, or partition, walls are installed and ceilings placed. This finishing separates the basement into enclosed spaces and introduces several problems.

Walls and ceilings can become musty in basements. Dividing the open basement into rooms blocks the healthful ventilation to these rooms. Air conditioned by the air exchanger and air conditioner may not supply fresh air to the basement, or it may be inadequate because the system was not designed to condition these new rooms. A dehumidifier placed in one enclosed area cannot dry the air trapped in other enclosed areas. In each enclosed room the air may be stagnant and humid and the contents of the room musty. My patients' symptoms grow steadily more severe.

During the life of your house your basement can and probably will flood; I believe that it is only a question of time before it happens. Once wet, all moldable items should be disposed of including the walls and ceilings that you installed with so much time and money. Once removed, do not replace them.

In a new home meticulously constructed for an allergic person by a skilled contractor, finishing the basement may be acceptable. Even in this new house, I would prefer that the entire area be open and the foundation walls accessible from inside the basement.

Dehumidifiers

Do not rely on the air conditioner to dry your house throughout the summer. It only dries the house on hot days when it is actively cooling the air. Also, with modern machines this cooling can be less than optimal and I will touch on this in the next chapter. Further, the air conditioner does not operate during the cool and often wet spring and fall. During these seasons, humidity accumulates in the basement. If the basement air is not dehumidified, the high humidity encourages the growth of mites and mold. Once established, these microorganisms continue to contaminate the home's air throughout the rest of the year, even in the winter. Therefore, neglecting summer dehumidification of the basement increases the mite and mold content of your home's air throughout the home, throughout the year.

Although I advise you to operate your dehumidifier continually from spring through late fall, I realize that on certain days it will not work efficiently. Dehumidifiers are normally designed for optimum efficiency at 80°F air temperature and 60 percent relative humidity. At normal room temperatures and humidity levels below 50 percent, their efficiency drops markedly. In spite of these defects, use yours throughout the summer anyway. Dehumidifiers work poorly in winter, as they tend to freeze up if the temperature is less than 65°F. Turn them off in winter if they freeze or stop dripping water into the pan. Alternatively, you can get models that are designed for operation at low temperatures.

How should you use the dehumidifier? I set mine to run continuously to keep the basement as dry as possible; the drier the air, the less mite and mold growth. When the dehumidifier pan is full it stops operating. To prevent you from forgetting to empty the full pan, run a hose from the outlet on the pan to the floor drain to provide for continuous drainage.

Continuous drainage into the floor drain also allows the dehumidifier to operate when you are away. It keeps the basement dry when the warm, pleasant summer breezes tempt you to shut off the air conditioner and open windows to let in this excellent air. To kill the germs that grow in the pan, hose, and drain, add three ounces of liquid bleach to the collecting pan once a week.

Do not think that a dehumidifier will allow you to have a dry carpet and pad in the basement. It won't. The carpet and pad on the concrete slab of the house cannot be dehumidified because the dehumidifier can only dry the air after humidity from the slab rises through the carpet and pad and enters the air above them. Even with a dehumidifier operating in the basement in summer, the humid microclimate in the carpet and pad will breed mites and mold there.

In new construction, proper building techniques reduce the amount of humidity in the basement and may make the continual operation of the dehumidifier less important. Comparatively few of these houses have been built and fewer aged for the years necessary to reveal hidden problems such as unexpected basement humidity, so I cannot offer any advice on these homes.

Storage in a Basement

Storing objects that can become moldy in a basement adds to the mold level in the basement and, because this air circulates throughout the house, the rest of the house. Do not store cardboard boxes in the basement as they can become moldy. Be careful of objects that can become musty such as magazines, blankets, clothes, and books; store them in airtight plastic containers. If you are a bookworm and like to save the books you read for a future reading, don't do it. Books can become moldy anywhere in a house but especially in the basement. It is best to dispose of books after you read them to keep them from accumulating in the house. If you must keep books, store them in airtight plastic containers.

Do not store firewood in the basement. This wood is moldy and will add to the moldiness of the house. Store it outside.

To assure good air circulation around and through the storage area, leave space between storage containers. Avoid enclosed storage areas that cannot be well ventilated, open these areas up to the ventilation provided by your cooled, cleaned, and refreshed air.

Laundry and Workbenches in Basements

You must approach clothes washing and drying with care, whether you locate the washer and dryer in the basement or on an upper floor. Assure good air circulation that quickly carries away washer moisture. The dryer must be vented to the outside—the warmed air emerging from these machines is very humid and contains yeast and other microorganisms. In addition, exhaust air from a gas dryer contains combustion gases, including carbon monoxide. Never dry clothes on a line in the basement; the wet clothes release too much humidity. Make sure there is a drain underneath the washer in case of overflow.

A workbench in the basement is acceptable, but dust-creating activities such as sawing and sanding should not be carried on in the house. Be careful to remove organic dusts such as sawdust as they can mold. A dirty workbench can be a source of mold; keep it clean.

Carpeting and Furniture in Basements

I will now return to the subject of carpet in the basement. I do so because it is such a potent source of the illnesses that plague my patients. Carpet collects the skin scales that all of us shed and form a nutrient bed where mites and mold grow. But mites and mold need more than this nutrient bed to grow; as we discussed, they need humidity levels in excess of 50 percent.

I have already mentioned—and now want to reemphasize—permanently placed carpet should not be in the basement. There, the carpet and pad rest on the slab of the house, a slab that continuously transmits the humidity of the ground into the house; it transmits this humidity throughout the year. The humidity grows mites and mold in carpet and pad throughout the year.

Throw or area rugs are acceptable. To destroy the dust mites that they harbor, several treatments are acceptable. Beating them while they hang on a line forcibly ejects mites and mold from the carpets. Freezing them by placing the rugs outside on a cold winter day works well. A third treatment relies on dust mites' high susceptibility to water loss, especially at higher temperatures. Placing the rugs in direct sunlight will simultaneously dry them and heat them, creating a microclimate hostile to mite survival. Simply "airing" them in temperatures that are neither freezing or drying does not kill mites.

The effect of these actions on mold is unknown, as I mentioned when we discussed mold. Therefore, it is best to try to control mold by keeping the rug dry and washing it in hot water.

Upholstered furniture should not be placed in a basement. The stuffing will in time harbor mites and become moldy. Although leather-covered furniture may be better than fabric-covered furniture, the stuffing will still become moldy and harbor mites.

Summary

You can see the importance I attach to a basement. It helps determine your health or illnesses. Because of its importance, let's review the above suggestions to help you find and maintain the best basement for your home.

I believe that the open basement without interior walls and ceilings is best. As the foundation walls are not hidden behind interior walls, they can be readily inspected for any leakage. Any water that gains entrance by rain, toilet overflow, or a leaking water pipe can be easily removed.

Walls and ceilings should not partition the various areas in the basement; they obstruct the airflow.

Make every effort to provide adequate, unencumbered, and continuous ventilation. With adequate ducts and air supplies in the basement, the air can be cooled by the air conditioner and refreshed by the air exchanger.

More can be done to keep the basement dry. When building a home, place a vapor barrier under the slab and waterproof or insulate the walls from the outside. Paint the inside walls with a vapor-retardant paint or sealer. If you must finish the floor, use tile, preferably ceramic tile, and cover it with throw rugs. Avoid crawl spaces; if one is present in the home, cover its floor with an efficient vapor barrier, or better yet, a vapor barrier topped with a concrete slab.

The basement should be free of upholstered furniture, cardboard boxes, and other objects that can become musty. Storage should be minimal and open, moldable items kept in plastic containers, and the storage units positioned so they won't block ventilation. A workbench and properly installed and vented washer and dryer are acceptable. Showers, hot tubs, and other humidity generators are not acceptable. Do not place a bedroom in the basement; if one has to be there, strictly follow the above advice and the advice on bedrooms that I will detail later in this book.

What You Want in a Basement

Feature	👍 Look for...	👎 Avoid...
Foundation	...a full basement extending under the entire house. ...a new home where proper steps have been taken to isolate the slab from ground moisture if slab construction is your only option. ...an enclosed crawl space with conditioned air, and that has a vapor barrier over the dirt and concrete over that if a house with a crawl space is your only option.	...a home with no basement. ...a slab-on-grade home where the slab is likely not water-proofed and will wick moisture into the living space. ...a crawl space that has an exposed dirt floor and is inadequately ventilated.
Moisture control	...a basement that has a properly installed vapor barrier under the slab, water-proofed walls, and a footing drain.	...a house without slab and foundation waterproofing. Note: Even new houses may have inadequate waterproofing. Verify with the builder which products were used.

Feature	👍 Look for...	👎 Avoid...
Air quality	...adequate supply of conditioned air from the home's HVAC ducts. Run a dehumidifier to help control moisture from spring through fall.	...damp, unventilated basements.
Garages	...an above-grade garage.	...tuck-under garages.
Finished living spaces	...unfinished space with exposed concrete walls and slab, and no partition walls or ceiling. ...sealed or painted concrete walls. ...bare, painted, or sealed concrete floors. Ceramic tile is acceptable, as are throw rugs. ...wood, metal, or plastic furniture (and only if furniture is necessary).	...a finished basement where wall coverings can hide leaking water and partition walls block airflow. ... any covering on the inside of a basement wall, other than sealer or paint. ...wall-to-wall carpet, wood, linoleum, vinyl, and plastic-laminate flooring. ...any upholstered furniture, even if leather- or plastic-covered.
Work spaces	...a properly drained and vented clothes washer and drier. ...a clean workbench and available space elsewhere for dust-making projects.	...venting the dryer into the basement. ...drying clothes on a line in the basement, which adds humidity. ...a dirty or dusty workbench.
Storage	...open storage units with adequate ventilation around them. ...airtight plastic storage containers for moldable fabric and paper products.	...enclosed, unventilated storage units. ...storing cardboard boxes in the basement. ...storing moldable items such as fabric and paper goods.

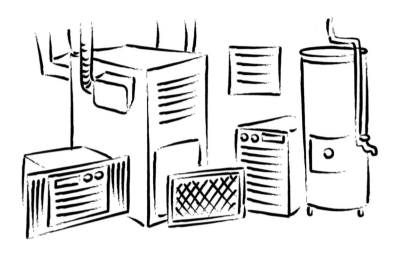

CHAPTER 5

The Appliances Circulating Air in Your Home

NOW THAT WE HAVE REVIEWED the largest potential for trouble in your home, let's move next to the appliances that can circulate air—bad and good—around your house. Proper attention to this equipment can significantly help improve your indoor air quality.

Combustion Appliances—Furnaces and Water Heaters

Combustion appliances, such as gas- or oil-fueled furnaces and water heaters, release harmful gases and particulates, plus moisture, as they burn fuel. To prevent these unhealthy by-products from entering the air in your home, your combustion appliances must be properly vented. Traditionally this was done simply by allowing the hot air to rise up the duct. Air to fuel the combustion came in through the various leaks in the home's exterior.

Today there are better options. Sealed-combustion appliances have intake and exhaust outlets connected directly to the outdoors. In newer, airtight homes this is important because appliances could otherwise draw air from sources such as chimneys. Power-vented appliances forcibly expel the combustion exhaust, although they still draw combustion air from within the home, making them second in preference to sealed-combustion appliances. Although sealed-combustion and power-vented appliances are more expensive, they keep the indoor air cleaner.

In the older house, make sure that you do not starve a furnace or water heater for air by enclosing it in a room without a vent. It will attempt to gain air for combustion by drawing it from the chimney and this is very dangerous.

I believe that the preferred energy for the furnace is natural gas. It burns cleaner than oil or wood. Wood-burning furnaces should be avoided as burning wood releases many pollutants that will gain entrance to the house when the furnace door is open, through any leaks in the exhaust ducts, or through windows or any air leaks in the walls after the smoke is discharged into the outside air. Also, any smoke-sensitive people living downwind from the wood-burning home will suffer from the smoke discharged by the wood furnace.

Air-Cleaning Options

Air filters can be separated into two categories: those located in the ducts of the house and those that are self-contained, portable machines used in individual rooms. In this section we will examine duct-mounted air cleaners, which are also called central air cleaners. Central air cleaners themselves can be separated into two categories: those that are placed into a slot in the ductwork and the more elaborate units that require special installation.

Flat Filters

Flat filters are the typical half- to one-inch-thick filters that fit into a slot between the furnace and the ductwork. These filters can be made of synthetic, cellulose, or glass fibers; foam; or slit or expanded aluminum that is either dry or coated with a viscous oil that traps particulates. These filters efficiently trap large particles but do a poor job of trapping the small (.3 to 10 micron diameter) particles that sink deeply into our lungs when we breathe them. The efficiency is increased somewhat when the filters contain fibers that have been permanently charged during manufacturing.

The following tips will help you select and maintain your furnace filter:

- Read the manufacturer's instructions on maintaining your furnace and how often a licensed heating contractor should inspect your furnace.

- Identify from the instructions the type of filter appropriate for your furnace. Select the highest-efficiency filter that your furnace accepts. (Look for the MERV rating that is usually listed on the packaging, the higher the better.)

- Replace your filter at the suggested intervals, usually about every three months. If you are introducing higher levels of particulates into your home by remodeling, burning candles, smoking tobacco, or other activities, replace the filter more often. Replace it more often if one of the occupants suffers from asthma, allergies, or other lung diseases.

Pleated Filters

Flat filters are poor at trapping bioaerosols because they cannot be packed full enough of particle-trapping fibers. Such tight packing would obstruct the flow of air through the filter and hence, through the ducts. To solve this problem, the efficiency is increased by packing more fibers of smaller diameter into the filter and then pleating it into an accordion shape. The pleats actually slow the air flow as it hits the filter and allow the air to work through the dense fibers, rather than bounce off the flat, dense surface. These filters are called extended-surface or pleated filters and can contain either charged or uncharged fibers.

While pleated filters are available to replace standard inch-thick furnace filters, a better option, I believe, is a thicker version that requires a special housing in the ductwork. Either way, pleated filters are a significant improvement over flat filters because they trap more of the fine particles and bioaerosols that we want to remove from the air.

High-Efficiency Particulate Air (HEPA) Filters

HEPA filters are a further improvement over extended-surface or pleated filters. The fibers in the HEPA filter are submicroscopic glass fibers that form a filter that looks and feels like blotter paper. The true HEPA filter requires so much pressure to force air through it that it is more suitable for industrial use than in the typical home. Thus, less dense and less-efficient filters called HEPA-type filters are available for the home. Although less efficient than true HEPA filters, they are far more efficient than flat or pleated filters. These filters need to be placed in a special housing in the ductwork that has a fan to assist air movement and a prefilter to extend their useful life.

Electronic Air Filters

Electronic filters use an electrical field to trap particles. Electronic precipitators are the most common type of electronic air cleaner. In the single-stage (and less efficient) design, a charged medium both charges air particles and collects them by attracting them to a medium having an opposite charge. A two-stage design is more effective. It charges incoming airborne particles using an electrode, or wire. The charged particles then enter a second stage, a series of oppositely charged metal plates. The charged particles precipitate on these plates, removing them from the air. The efficiency of these filters varies depending on air flow, surface area of the plates, and the strength of the electrical field.

The negative ion generator is a simpler form of electronic air cleaner. It induces a static charge on the air particles, which are then attracted to and deposited on surfaces in the room, including walls, ceilings, tabletops, curtains, and occupants. Promoters of these devices often claim that the ions change fumes and smoke to render them less harmful or to force them out of the air. The use of these machines is very controversial, with many studies showing that they produce ozone and are not as effective as claimed.

An important point to keep in mind when selecting a filter is that efficiency will change over time. As panel, pleated, and HEPA filters become loaded with particles, the available openings for air to flow through become smaller. The result is better filtration but less air movement, causing your furnace to work harder to move air through the system. You must replace the filters regularly, which can be expensive.

Electronic precipitators are most efficient when first installed and lose their efficiency as they get dirty. Although they do not need to be replaced, regular maintenance and cleaning is required to keep electronic precipitators operating at peak efficiency.

In the home of the allergic person, I recommend installing either an electrostatic precipitator or a HEPA filter in the heating and air conditioning ducts. They generally attain greater efficiency than pleated or panel filters for capturing dust particles that are of such small size that they can be breathed into the lung.

Note: Relying on the central air cleaner to clean the air of the musty home, instead of correcting the conditions that cause mustiness, is a great mistake. The musty home generates mite and mold allergens faster than the central air cleaner can remove them. Furthermore, central air cleaners are limited; they remove only some of allergens floating in home air—those that are light enough to float for such prolonged periods that they can reach the filter. Thus they give only partial relief of allergic symptoms sparked by contaminating bioaerosols. They cannot clean the air of heavy contaminants—such as heavy mold particles and dust mite feces—that fall out of the air quickly; these particles do not float in the air long enough to reach the central air cleaner.

Should You Consider Air Duct Cleaning?

The worth of this procedure is uncertain. There may be value in ridding the ducts of construction debris. One study reported by researcher Amy Tsay at the Academy of Allergy, Asthma and Immunology annual meeting in 2001 found that ducts that deliver conditioned air throughout a house are almost free of substances that cause allergic reactions. Their conclusion, "Air duct cleaning appears to be of limited value in reducing animal allergen levels in homes, and would not be recommended as a method for controlling mite allergen exposure."

If air ducts must be insulated, be sure that the insulation is on the outside of the ducts so that dusts and microorganisms cannot accumulate there.

Furnace-Mounted Humidifiers

Pumping moisture into the winter home through a central humidifier moistens irritated nasal mucus membranes (the inner lining of the nose and throat), which is comforting. However, a furnace-mounted humidifier also increases the humidity level in the home and fosters higher levels of mites and mold. Trying to combat the winter nasal dryness through higher home humidity may be an effort doomed to failure. My experience in treating allergy patients convinces me that the irritating dryness of the nose and throat suffered in the winter home comes not from house dryness but from breathing excess levels of molds and mite.

Mites and mold can only be defeated in a dry home. Prompting their growth by raising the home's humidity with a central humidifier provokes more nasal irritation and induces or worsens symptoms caused by high levels of mites and mold: headaches, cough, incessant colds, repeated nasal and sinus infections, and recurrent pneumonia. (An exception to this thought is the person who suffers because of a medical condition that causes dryness of the mucus membranes. Check with your medical professional.)

I tell my patients to disconnect the furnace humidifier. If fine furniture or woodwork will be ruined by the resulting dryness, they have to make a choice between the furniture/woodwork and their health. If they complain that the dryness causes sparks when they touch objects, I tell them to moisten the house when the sparks jump from you to an object on the wall when you are standing in the middle of a room. A bit ludicrous, but it helps stress the point.

Air Exchangers

For people with allergies, the air exchanger is the most important air-handling machine to install in home. It continually brings fresh air into the home while exhausting the stale air trapped inside. It accomplishes this by drawing fresh outside air into the home through one duct and expelling stale indoor air through another duct. Why not just open the window? Although opening a window does allow fresh air to enter the house, it does not distribute it evenly throughout the house. Individual areas containing stale, musty air may not be ventilated. Only by distributing fresh air through a properly designed duct system can a whole house be properly ventilated.

When cold outside air is introduced into a house and heated by the house air, its relative humidity is reduced; it can absorb the humidity generated in generous quantities by our daily activities. (For example, outside air at -22°F and 100 percent relative humidity when heated to 68°F will have a relative humidity of less than 2 percent. This dry air can dry your home!) The constant replacement of humid inside air with dry outside air carries away moisture; the higher the air replacement rate, the lower the humidity level.

HRV or ERV?

There are presently two types of air exchangers being regularly installed. The Heat Recovery Ventilator (HRV) is typically installed only in cold-climate homes. In winter the HRV removes heat from outgoing house air and uses that energy to warm the cold incoming outdoor air. In summer the process is reversed, with heat being removed from the incoming air and transferred to the outgoing air. The HRV does not, however, transfer moisture from one air stream to the other.

If an HRV is not controlled by a thermostat that is adjusted for the outside temperature, be sure that you change the temperature setting to reflect the temperature of the outside air. Not changing this setting is the most frequent mistake HRV owners make. In summer, to allow the air conditioner and dehumidifier to dry the house on humid days, it is best to turn off the air exchanger, as it will draw in too much humid air for these other machines to dry. Some models have controls that adjust for humid summer weather and do not need this constant changing.

The Energy Recovery Ventilator (ERV), on the other hand, exchanges both heat and moisture and is suited for use in most of the U.S. In winter it removes heat and humidity from the outgoing air and returns it to the incoming air. In summer it removes the heat and humidity from the incoming air and transfers it to the outgoing air. Note that while preserving the indoor humidity in cold winter climates may be considered by builders to be good for the health of the house itself, it defeats the goal of allergy sufferers to maintain the low humidity levels that kill mites and mold!

The Benefits of an Air Exchanger

The air exchanger is a must for the modern, tightly insulated home where trapped air accumulates humidity arising from cooking, cleaning, laundry, bathing, and breathing (our breath is very humid). This humidity can penetrate through the house walls, reaching the barrier that wraps around the house, the barrier that prevents air from gaining entrance to the house. If the outside temperature is low, it can then condense on this barrier and in the cool walls behind the barrier. This condensed humidity turns to water, rotting the walls and immeasurably worsening the air quality. A well-functioning air exchanger, by keeping the house air dry, resists this harmful condensation at the outside walls.

The air exchanger also expels fumes generated by construction material, new carpeting, cleaning fluids, perfumes, and other fume-generating sources. I believe an air exchanger is also a great help to the older home where age has allowed the home to become musty.

While an air exchanger does take energy—and money—to run, it recoups some of these costs by preconditioning the incoming air.

A Balanced System

To properly vent a house, all rooms the size of a walk-in closet or greater must have both supply and return vents. If the room has only supply vents, the air supplied by these supply vents cannot readily escape from the room. The room will be inadequately vented.

The supply and exhaust of an air exchanger must be carefully calibrated. I like the idea of maintaining a very slight positive air pressure in the house, which tends to resist movement of allergens into the house, "pushing" them out. However, if there is too great a positive pressure in the house, it can force moisture into the walls, leading to rot problems. Avoid creating negative air pressure in the house. This can starve combustion appliances such as gas stoves and fireplaces of the air they need, creating a potentially dangerous situation called back drafting. We will return to these combustion devices later.

To help the air exchanger operate properly, all joints in the ductwork must be properly sealed with mastic, or mastic and mesh tape in areas subject to vibration. (Ironically, while duct tape will hold together just about anything else you apply it too, it's actually not a good choice for sealing ducts.) Unsealed ductwork leaks air. These leaks may allow negative pressure to build up in the basement and suck humid air into the basement. This air condenses on the cool foundation walls, promoting the growth of mold.

What about the Bath and Kitchen Fans?

Whether you still need bathroom fans will depend on the installation of the air exchanger. If the air exchanger shares the HVAC ductwork and there are supplies and returns in the bathrooms, the air exchanger can take care of bathroom humidity. If it is on a stand-alone ducting system, or it's been retrofitted in an older house that doesn't have vents in the bathroom—or if the air exchanger is an HRV used only in winter—you will still need separate bath vents to exhaust humidity from showering and bathing.

Regardless of how the air exchanger is installed, you will still need a vent fan in the kitchen to remove vaporized grease, combustion by-products, and other air contaminants generated by cooking.

Which Appliance is Most Important for the Allergy Sufferer?

The air exchanger is so important that, if homeowner funds are limited, they should first be spent to buy a dehumidifier for the basement; second, to install an air exchanger; and third, to place an air conditioner in the room of the hay fever sufferer. Only after these machines are installed should central air cleaning be added to the heating and cooling ducts.

Studies support my belief. Homes with air exchangers have been shown to have significantly lower humidity levels than those without an exchanger. These studies also show that at the same time that the air exchanger decreases the humidity, it also decreases mite numbers in mite hideouts such as mattresses and carpets in the ventilated areas of the homes, as well as reducing animal hair, dander, and saliva.

The Central Air Conditioner

Every home with an allergy sufferer should have a central air conditioner. When summer's pollen and high mold levels cause sneezing, wheezing, and other miseries, the air conditioned home is a welcome refuge—closing the windows denies entrance of pollen and mold into the home. While the system actively cools the air, it also removes much of the high humidity that discomforts the homeowner and prompts mite and mold growth.

There is a problem, however, and it concerns the newer air conditioners. The older central air conditioners briefly cooled the air below the temperature needed to maintain comfort. This extra cooling removed large quantities of water and resulted in lower humidity. Unfortunately, the newer central air conditioners cool the air to just below the required temperature; without this extra cooling jolt they remove less humidity.

To help this situation, whole-house dehumidifiers have been developed to dry the air to a humidity level less than that needed to propagate mites and mold. They are expensive but may be affordable when building a new house. If you do not have this new system installed, and if your basement is poorly ventilated by the existing ductwork, on humid days continue to run a freestanding dehumidifier in the basement at the same time you operate the air conditioner.

Now that we have looked at the appliances that help keep us comfortable, let's look at the place where we receive the most comfort in our house—the bedroom.

What You Want in Air-Conditioning Appliances

Appliance	👍 Look for...	👎 Avoid...
Furnace and water heater	...natural gas or electric appliances. ...sealed combustion or power venting. ...a dedicated source of combustion air.	...oil- or wood-burning units. ...furnaces or water heaters in an enclosed space without an air source.
Air cleaners	...a furnace-mounted HEPA or electrostatic precipitator air cleaner. ...pleated and/or charged media filters if the above are not an option.	...a home without ductwork as there is no way to centrally clean the air. ...improperly functioning electronic filters as they can emit harmful ozone.
Central humidifier	...a house without a central humidifier so that dry air can kill mites and mold	....a central humidifier (unless medically necessary). They promote mite and mold growth.
Air exchanger	...a properly installed and balanced HRV or ERV, especially in new, airtight construction where moisture problems are common.	...an improperly installed system that is unbalanced as it may actually create moisture problems or cause combustion appliances to back draft.

Appliance	Look for...	⬇ Avoid...
Air conditioner	...a central air conditioner with supplementary dehumidification if necessary.	...a home without central AC. The high cost of installing and running air conditioning and dehumidification equipment is offset by money saved on medicines, doctors, and lost workdays.

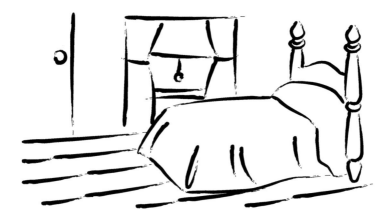

CHAPTER 6

The Bedroom: Your Refuge from Allergies

WE DISCUSSED HOW THE BASEMENT is a major determinant of your health or illnesses. If you live in or above a musty basement, you will find it hard to be healthy. Another area of your home that also determines your health or illness is the bedroom. If properly set up, it provides a refuge, a reprieve from the dust mite, mold, and animal allergens that you must face daily at home, at work, in school, and in the other places you visit during the day.

Think of your bedroom as a hospital where you can recover from the stuffiness, wheezing, headaches, and other illnesses brought by allergic exposures. You spend a significant part of each day there, from four to ten hours—and these hours in your one-room hospital can help heal you. The allergy-free hours you spend there prepare you to face the next day more resistant to the allergic exposures you will encounter. The more severe your symptoms, the more carefully you should prepare your bedroom as a refuge.

As we examine various aspects of the bedroom we will follow the recommendations—with some modification—of the National Institute of Allergy and Infectious Diseases, National Institutes of Health.

Location of the Bedroom

The best location for a bedroom is on the second floor of a home, separated from the basement by the first floor. The next best location is on the first floor. Locating a bedroom in the basement is a mistake—the basement is the mustiest area of a home. I have often seen patients' health improve significantly when they leave the basement bedroom for a bedroom on the first or second floor. If the bedroom must be in the basement, closely follow all the environmental suggestions in this book to prepare this room for the allergic person.

It can be argued that a bedroom can be placed in the basement of a home built with good vapor barriers protecting the basement from humidity. As these home are still relatively new and long-term problems unknown, I would not advise placing the bedroom in the basement of these homes until we know more about them.

Carpet

We discussed carpets when we discussed the basement. They trap dust and serve as home to dust mites, mold, and animal dander—they make controlling these allergens difficult. We will discuss carpets and pads further when we examine the first and second floor of the house. For now it is sufficient to note that in a bedroom that you want to make a refuge from the allergens you face daily, carpet and pad are not acceptable. Keeping carpets out of bedrooms is truly effective in maintaining a low-allergen room. Studies show that low bedroom allergen levels were found in bedrooms with no carpet even when adjacent rooms were carpeted.

The Bed, Mattress, and Pillow

It is best to have only one bed in the bedroom. Encase its box spring in a vinyl or plastic casing. Encase the mattress and pillow in a dust- or allergen-proof cover made of tightly woven, breathable fabric. This prevents dust-containing mite and mold allergens from being forced from the mattress and pillows and drawn into your nose and lungs as you sleep.

When buying a cloth cover, examine it closely to make sure that it is tightly woven. Scientists have measured how tightly cloth needs to be woven to form an effective barrier. They found that dust mite allergens are blocked from exiting from the mattress and pillow by a pore size of less than 10 μm (micrometers). The mites themselves are blocked by a pore size of 20 μm, the width of the larval stage. As the mite larvae are usually greater than 50 μm across, a cover with a pore size of less than 20 μm will prevent mites from entering a pillow or mattress.

Tip: In winter, when temperatures are below freezing, placing mattresses and pillows outside for twenty-four hours kills the mites they contain.

A feather pillow with a tightly woven cover is probably better than a synthetic pillow, which harbors mites. As an added precaution, I recommend you replace pillows every two years. If the bed has exposed bedsprings, scrub them outside the room. If a second bed must be in the room, prepare it in the same manner.

Bedding

The choice of blankets and other bedding material can make the difference between a peaceful night's sleep or a troubled sleep with nasal stuffiness and morning headaches. Avoid fuzzy wool blankets or down comforters. Use a Dacron mattress pad. Use only washable materials on the bed. Wash bedding (sheets, blankets, and other bedclothes) weekly in water that is at least 130°F (55°C): this temperature kills dust mites and removes their allergens. It probably also kills mold. I do not recommend washing pillows, especially feather pillows, which may not dry thoroughly in the dryer, allowing mold to grow in the moist interior. Some synthetic pillows, however, are designed to withstand machine washing and drying; check the manufacturer's instructions. Finally, some drycleaners do clean pillows, although the chemicals may affect some allergy suffers. Perhaps the safest course of all is to avoid cleaning pillows at all and replace them periodically.

If you set your hot water temperature at a lower temperature (which is commonly done to prevent children from scalding themselves), wash bedding at a commercial establishment that uses high water temperatures. Alternatively, adding benzyl benzoate (0.03 percent) and eucalyptus oil (0.2 percent) to the wash cycle also kills mites, but the oil leaves an odor in the bedclothes for two to three days. These products are available from companies that specialize in products for allergy sufferers.

Tumble drying blankets kills all mites if a temperature greater than 130°F is maintained for ten minutes. Dry cleaning kills all mites but does not remove all their allergens.

Humidifiers and Vaporizers

When I first opened my allergy office, the number of patients I was asked to treat who suffered severe asthma surprised me. I became a local hero for the marvelous relief I gave these pitiable sufferers. My secret? I turned off all of their vaporizers and humidifiers!

But, before they would turn off their vaporizers and humidifiers, I had to answer an objection each patient raised. Doesn't increased humidity moisten the nose and throat and lungs? Isn't it healthy? The answer is: Yes and no. Yes, it does moisten the nose and throat. No, it is not healthy. As I mentioned, I believe that dry nose and throat is not caused by low humidity, but by breathing irritating bioaerosols. Your nose and throat feel this irritation as dryness and your attempt to moisten the air to combat this perceived dryness only adds to the mite and mold contamination of the air, worsening your feeling of dryness.

A humidifier is not necessary to moisten the air reaching the lungs. Our noses and large air passages humidify the air as it passes through the respiratory tract before it reaches the lung. A humidifier does not increase this humidity. Any gains conferred by humidifiers and vaporizers are offset by their generation of bioaerosols.

Humidifiers are such a common source of the harmful bioaerosols that doctors now diagnose these illnesses as *humidifier fever*. Protozoa, mold, amoebas, and strains of bacteria have been found in humidifiers; they are readily released into the air as the humidifier releases its moisture. These germs make people sick. Further, they generate the high humidity that prompts mite and mold growth on nearby walls and ceilings, in carpets, pads, upholstered furniture, and beds. People who use humidifiers and vaporizers are living in the humidity and mold of a rain forest.

If you must humidify because you or a family member has a cough or sore throat, use a vaporizer, use it for no more than two hours, and wash it out with soap and water before the next use. Never use a humidifier.

Note: If you have a medical condition that requires use of a humidifier or vaporizer, you will have to disregard this advice.

More Information About Bedrooms

A discussion of the bedroom would be incomplete without mentioning the following typical bedroom contents and cleaning methods for the bedroom.

Pets and Plants

We will discuss pets in a later chapter, here I give you this caution: Keep all pets out of the room. If you must keep an aquarium, do not put it in the bedroom. Keep no plants in the bedrooms. Experience has taught me that close exposure to the wet dirt in plants increases congestion, wheezing, and headaches. And artificial plants are simply dust catchers.

Furniture and Furnishings

Go for the minimalist look. Avoid upholstered furniture and venetian blinds. A wooden, plastic, or metal chair that can be scrubbed may be used in the bedroom. If desired, hang plain, lightweight curtains on the windows. It's a common misconception that blinds—whether wood, metal, or vinyl—are better for allergy sufferers than fabric curtains, which can harbor mites. However, fabric curtains can be washed, while blinds can be very difficult to clean thoroughly. Wash the curtains weekly with the bedclothes at 130°F.

Cleaning

Clean the room once a week, taking pains to clean thoroughly and completely. Clean the floors, furniture, tops of doors, window frames, sills, etc., with a damp cloth or oil mop (a damp cloth catches dust while a dry cloth simply stirs it up); air the room thoroughly; then close the doors and windows until the dust-sensitive person is ready to occupy the room. Be sure to clean under the bed.

Tip: A cleaning service I know of that specializes in cleaning for allergy sufferers uses a high-quality, portable HEPA air cleaner that they move from room to room as they clean. It helps catch any dust that does get stirred up while cleaning.

Air Cleaners

I believe that both central and freestanding room air cleaners have a place in the home of the allergy sufferer. I discussed central air cleaners in Chapter Five. A room air cleaner supplements a central air cleaner by helping to free the air of dust mite allergens and the mold particles that are too heavy to reach the central air cleaner. This air cleaner should be the HEPA-type unit. Avoid ionizing air cleaners in the bedroom—the ozone they produce is troublesome.

Dehumidifiers

First and second floor bedrooms should not need dehumidifiers. If the house has a basement bedroom, a dehumidifier should be located close to the bedroom and the door left open so the bedroom air is continually dried. Care should be taken to clean the unit frequently to prevent mold growth.

Toys

Try to keep toys that will accumulate dust or become musty out of the bedroom. Avoid stuffed toys or keep their numbers small and wash them with the bedclothes. Freeze soft toys for twenty-four hours—either in the freezer or outdoors in freezing weather—to kill mites, then wash them to remove mite allergens. Washable toys of wood, rubber, metal, or plastic are acceptable, but do not allow them to clutter a room and become dust catchers.

Clothes

Start by emptying and cleaning all closets and, if possible, storing their contents elsewhere. To retard mustiness, all closets, whether on the upper floors or in the basement, should have louvered doors or be left open to allow air conditioned, cleaned, and refreshed house air to enter. It is best to keep clothing in zippered plastic bags and shoes in racks or in plastic containers.

Reflections

The bedroom is your hospital room, your retreat from the allergens that make your nose and chest stuffy, your skin itch, your head hurt, your refuge from the allergens that depress your immune system, forcing you to suffer colds and sinus infections. The more severely you are affected, the more compulsively you should dust- and moisture-proof your bedroom.

The actions that I discussed may seem difficult at first. However, experience plus habit will make them easier. The results—better breathing, fewer medications, and greater freedom from allergy and asthma attacks—are well worth the effort.

In the next chapter, we will leave the bedroom and look at ideas for making the rest of the house healthy.

What You Want in a Bedroom

Feature	👍 Look for...	👎 Avoid...
Location in the house	...a bedroom on the second floor. The first floor will do if there is no alternative.	...a basement bedroom.
Floor covering	...hardwood, tile, or resilient flooring. Throw rugs that you can beat with a carpet beater, expose to the drying sun or freezing air, or wash in hot water are acceptable.	...wall-to-wall carpeting.
Mattresses and pillows	...tightly woven coverings for box springs, mattresses, and pillows. ...feather pillows unless you are allergic to them.	...older, unencased mattresses. ...unencased synthetic pillows.
Bedding	...synthetic blankets, Dacron mattress pads, and cotton sheets that can withstand frequent washing at high temperatures.	...fuzzy blankets and down comforters. ...infrequent washing of bedding. ...washing bedding in temperatures less than 130°F.
Humidity	...a home with a good air-handling system so the use of a humidifier or vaporizer is unnecessary.	...using a humidifier or vaporizer in a bedroom unless medically necessary.

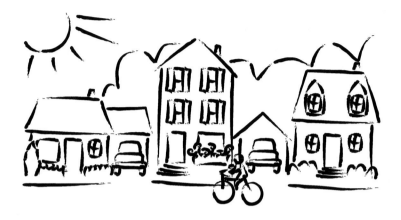

CHAPTER 7

The First and Second Floors
of the House

WE HAVE LOOKED AT THE BASEMENT and the bedroom and discussed how to keep them as free of allergens as possible. Now we will see what actions we can take to reduce the allergy potential of the first and second floor of the home. As I discuss the first and second floor I will return to the subject of floor covering. As we are not dealing with the basement or the bedroom, there is more freedom in our choices. If you place carpets on these floors, you need some guidance on how to care for them and I will discuss this care.

The kitchen stove is usually on these floors, as are showers, baths, and fireplaces; I will comment on them and on the need for good air supply to these areas. Finally I will mention painting and wallpapering walls, and comment on keeping books and plants in the house.

Carpets

When we examined the basement, I noted that carpet and pad used in a basement rest on the concrete slab of the house. Throughout the year, this slab transfers humidity from the ground into the carpet and pad. This humidity promotes troubling mold and mite growth in carpet and pad in summer and, because the slab is moist throughout the year, mite and mold grow there even in winter. Therefore, permanently placed carpets and pads should not be in the basement except perhaps in the case of the new home with proper vapor barriers.

In the home with a basement extending under the whole house, the basement serves as an air space that separates the first floor from the slab. Because this air space separates the first floor from this humid slab, carpet placed the first or second floor does not have the same potential to pick up moisture from the slab. In winter, in temperate climates, carpet is generally not subjected to the 50 percent humidity necessary for abundant mite and mold growth. Even in tightly insulated homes, the air exchanger prevents home air from becoming stale and humid in winter. In summer this dryness is maintained by the air conditioner during humid days—the air conditioner reduces the humidity in the air that reaches the carpet.

Therefore, in the home with air conditioning and an air exchanger, carpet on the first and second floor should be acceptable as long as it is in good shape and not too old. Carpet on the first and second floor that has been contaminated by pets or exposed to excess moisture by vaporizers or humidifiers should be removed. Removal should also be considered in the tightly insulated modern home that does not have an air exchanger as its excessive high humidity over several winters may make the carpet and pad musty.

Steam cleaning usually does not penetrate deeply enough into the carpet and pad to remove the large numbers of mites and mold that live there. The water that remains after steam cleaning promotes more mite and mold growth, leaving the carpet and pad even more contaminated than they were before the cleaning. Keep the carpets clean and replace them when they become too old or too dirty. Carpets that have been subjected to repeated steam cleaning should be removed.

Note that the above does not apply if the main living areas of the house rest directly on the concrete slab of the building. In this case the living areas should be treated as I described in the chapter on basements.

Treating Carpet to Kill Dust Mites

Benzyl benzoate is often used to kill dust mites in carpet, but is it effective and safe? Used properly, it is safe. Benzyl benzoate is nontoxic, safe enough to use as a preservative in human food, and licensed to be painted on the skin of children. There are no reports of toxicity despite widespread use in homes. It is also effective as a scabicide—a substance to kill dust mites—in the laboratory.

But, does it effectively kill mites living in sofas or carpets with their large accumulations of human detritus? Some researchers do not believe it is possible to introduce sufficient quantities of benzyl benzoate into dirty carpet or carpet with heavy pile to be effective. If it is effective, finer powders may be the most effective preparation.

Tannic acid, a denaturing or protein-disrupting agent used to tan leather, is another product used for treating carpet. It has very low oral toxicity. In fact, we drink it in large quantities when we drink tea. However, it has a weakness when used to denature mites: It also denatures other proteins in carpet or dust so its activity can be used up before it degrades all the mite protein in the carpet. Homes that contain a cat will have such a huge quantity of cat protein that other proteins, including the protein from mites, will be inadequately treated. At present, the enthusiasm for routine use of this agent is limited.

Whether either of these agents are truly useful is questionable. Unquestionable is the very real possibility that using them will lull the homeowner into the belief that he can keep a carpet that should not be in the house. Further, the pad, which can be moldy and mite filled, is not affected by these agents.

Vacuuming and Dusting

Be sure to vacuum and dust the house weekly. When dusting use a cloth that absorbs dust instead of stirring it into the air. Wear a dust mask and leave the room for twenty minutes after cleaning to let the dust settle. An air cleaner will help remove allergens that escape into the air while you dust and vacuum.

The choice of a vacuum is critical. Ordinary vacuum cleaners and vacuum cleaner bags release large quantities of dust mite, mold, and pet protein back into the air. High-quality vacuum cleaners and vacuum cleaner bags release less of these allergens and help allergic people by reducing the amount of allergen they breathe. A number of vacuum cleaners on the market today claim to capture 99.9 percent of the tiny particles that can penetrate to the lungs when you breathe them.

Testing of different vacuum cleaner bags showed that high-quality three-layer bags (referred to as microfiltration bags) were the vacuum bags most effective in stopping allergen leakage, with two-layer bags being less effective. In contrast, single-thickness bags allowed far more allergens to pass through the machine and into the air. Vacuum cleaners with HEPA filters were effective in reducing the allergens liberated from the carpet while cleaning.

The best way to avoid breathing allergens stirred up by the vacuum cleaner is to install a central vacuum system that vents its exhaust to the outside.

The Kitchen Stove

I discourage the installation and use of gas stoves because burning gas releases pollution into the kitchen. Natural gas, composed of methane, impurities, and odorant, contains pollutant chemicals that can increase allergy symptoms and increase the symptoms suffered by people sensitive to airborne chemicals. Its combustion gases, unburned fuel, and chemical additives can be major sources of indoor air pollution.

Researchers say adult asthmatics who cook regularly on gas stoves are about twice as likely to receive emergency room treatment for asthma. The findings are the latest in a series of studies that suggest a link between gas stoves and respiratory problems. Every kitchen should have an exhaust fan to expel combustion by-products (if there is a gas range) and the grease and food particles created by cooking.

It is preferable to install a fan that vents to the outdoors. Recirculating fans do trap some grease in their filters, but do nothing to eliminate the combustion by-products created by a gas range.

Fireplaces

Although beautiful, fireplaces can discharge a lot of pollution into the home from burning gas or wood. In addition, downdrafts can release foul-smelling odors into the house. If you have a fireplace, install an insert that tightly seals the fireplace to prevent these gases and odors from gaining access to your home. In new homes, code usually requires that gas fireplaces be sealed-combustion units vented to the outside, a most favorable stipulation. These fireplaces are also very energy-efficient. Some areas still allow wood-burning fireplaces. If you have one, I recommend installing doors and a top-mounted damper to keep pollutants out of your home and increase its energy-efficiency.

Balancing Exhaust Fans

Most homes will have exhaust fans in the bathrooms and the kitchen. They may also have gas appliances (furnace, water heater, and fireplace) that consume air as they burn fuel. All of these appliances require a source of makeup air or they can create negative pressure in the home, causing air to be drawn in through the walls or even down the chimney and appliance vents. This danger is especially acute if the homeowners use an oversized kitchen vent fan or an unsealed fireplace.

The kitchen vent fan will remove a large quantity of air from the house. The air moved by a fan is measured in cubic feet per minute, or cfm. To help you visualize the volume of air a fan removes from the house, think of the volume of one cubic foot as equal to four footballs. Therefore, a 200–600 cfm stove exhaust fan will remove air equivalent to 800–2400 footballs of air per minute.

To replace this great volume of air, be sure that you have a ready source of makeup air, such as properly functioning air exchanger. It can supply replacement air to the tightly sealed home. Otherwise, as mentioned above, running the fan creates negative pressure that can cause spillage from older draft-vented combustion appliances (i.e. the gases don't exit up the chimney, but are drawn throughout the house), creating a dangerous situation.

It's also worth noting that code regulates where exhaust ducts can exit the house in order to avoid drawing exhaust air out of one outlet and in through one next to it if negative pressure is created inside the house.

In new construction the homeowner should obtain written proof from contractors and installers that the home has a plentiful supply of air to allow the fans to work properly and safely. In this newly constructed home, a properly installed air exchanger removes the need to vent the bathroom and shower to the outside, avoiding the need to perforate the walls of the house to install these vents.

Showers and Bathrooms

Showers and bathrooms are a potent source of the bioaerosols we are trying to reduce. Mold and mildew often build up in showers and tubs, along wall surfaces (particularly in corners and where the floor meets the wall), on the ceiling, and in the vanity area. Combat them by regularly using a mildew remover. Some tub-and-tile cleaners are meant to be sprayed on the surfaces of the shower and tub following each use, helping to prevent the accumulation of mold and mildew. If water from the shower gains entrance to the walls around it or floor beneath it, it can rot them and all this rotted material must be removed.

Showers in basements add to the mustiness of a basement and should not be there. Wherever they are situated, in the older house they should be vented to the outside and the vent fan turned on while showering and bathing to remove the humid air. In new homes with adequate ventilation, they should be continually ventilated by the central air ducts, dispersing the humidity generated by bathing and showering; this ventilation is especially necessary if the rooms do not have vents to the outside, as is currently recommended.

One-piece shower enclosures are preferred for the home of the allergic person as they are easier to clean and do not harbor mold as tile and shower curtains do. Cement backer board should back the shower surround, not moisture-resistant drywall. The base of the shower should be made of molded fiberglass.

If your shower and tub surround are tiled, cement backer board is the substrate of choice because it doesn't disintegrate when moistened. Moisture-resistant drywall, or greenboard, is not water-resistant. It is still commonly used as a tile substrate, but it shouldn't be. It gets soggy when wet, causing more grout cracks, causing more water seepage, causing more sogginess, and round and round it goes. Moisture-resistant drywall cannot be applied over a vapor barrier. If it is, any moisture that seeps through the grout effectively becomes trapped in the greenboard, hastening its demise.

All grout will allow some moisture to wick through. Like any concrete product, that's the nature of the beast. That's why choice of substrate is so important. That's also why many installers go for the safe option of installing a prefab shower base with tile walls. If you prefer a custom shower with a tile base, it is a must to have a professional tilesetter float a mortar bed and carefully install a suitable pan, usually fabricated from a single piece of EPDM rubber. It runs six to eight inches up the walls and is carefully cemented around the drain, leaving the weep holes exposed. Care is taken to avoid puncturing it. All of these precautions are necessary to prevent water from seeping through the base and rotting the subfloor and floor joists below.

Sealing grout only makes it resistant to staining—it retards, but does not prevent, moisture seepage. Latex-fortified grouts are stronger and more resistant to moisture and cracking and are becoming the standard. Intact grout joints on walls are usually not a seepage problem as the water runs rapidly down the walls. The joints in the floor are not an issue as long as the pan is properly sloped toward the drain and the pan is prepared as above.

One big culprit for water damage, however, is failing grout joints: cracked, flaking, and missing grout allows water behind the tiles. If you have damaged grout, it must be scraped out with a grout saw and replaced (if the tile is all still firmly attached). Inspect grout joints quarterly and do maintenance as soon as you see it is needed.

Caulk, and the lack thereof, is the other big culprit in bathroom moisture problems. Caulk must be applied anywhere two different planes meet: floor and wall, wall and wall, wall and ceiling, wall and tub, tub and floor. Grout in these joints will fail, guaranteed. Caulk should be inspected quarterly to make sure it is still intact. If not, it must be removed and reapplied. This caulking advice goes for solid-surface and fiberglass or acrylic surrounds, as well. Anywhere two planes meet and there is water involved, you must be vigilant with the caulk.

Paint and Wallcoverings

Vapor impermeable wallcoverings or paint will block the movement of vapor from the walls into the home. Moisture will accumulate behind the wallcovering or paint and grow mold. Make sure that your wallcovering and paint is vapor permeable, that it allows this moisture to pass through into the house where your ventilation equipment can dispose of it.

Plants in the Home

Wet dirt in the pots that contain plants supports a rich growth of microorganisms. My experience with patients shows me that having too many plants in a home adversely affects the health of the home's occupants. To keep the wet dirt in your house to an acceptable level, keep no more than four to five plants in the house.

Books in the Home

As I mentioned when I discussed basements, do not accumulate shelves of books. They become moldy easily. If you must keep some books, keep only a small number and keep them out of the basement. Any books in the basement not stored in airtight plastic containers should be discarded because they are probably already moldy.

The Importance of Being Careful

You may not believe that you need to be so careful in constructing or maintaining a home. One of the ways I can show you that you need to take this care—that your actions will determine your health—is to tell you stories about my patients. They learned the importance of being careful. We will look at the stories of some of my other patients in the following chapter.

What You Want in Living Areas

Feature	👍 Look for...	👎 Avoid...
Floor covering	...hard surfaces such as wood, tile, vinyl, and plastic-laminate flooring, although clean, well-maintained carpet is acceptable if the main floor is not on the concrete slab.	...carpet that is old, has been exposed to excessive humidity, or has pet damage. ...wood flooring or carpet applied to a concrete slab. ...carpet in bedrooms.
Carpet cleaning	...a central vacuum system that collects dust in a bin located in the garage or basement. A vacuum with a HEPA filter and/or micro-filtration bags is a good alternative.	...using vacuums with single-layer bags; they release too much allergenic material back into the air. ...repeated steam-cleaning of carpets.
Kitchen appliances	...an electric range with a properly sized and vented exhaust fan. ...an adequate supply of makeup air for the home's exhaust fans.	...gas ranges and kitchens without exhaust fans.
Bathrooms	...a properly sized exhaust fan to remove humidity caused by showering and bathing. ...well-maintained grout and caulk around the tub and shower.	...bathrooms that lack ventilation adequate to remove humidity that can lead to growth of mites and mold. ...deteriorated grout and caulk that allow water to collect in the walls, leading to rot and mold.
Wall-coverings	...permeable paint and wall-coverings that allow moisture to dissipate.	...impermeable paint and wall-coverings that can trap moisture behind them.

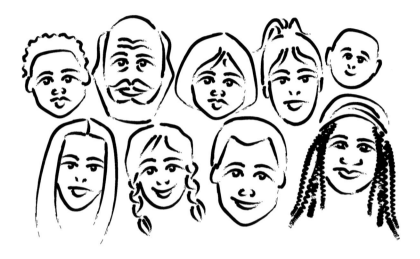

CHAPTER 8

Patients Whose Homes
Made Them Sick

AT THIS STAGE IN OUR DISCUSSION, you may be getting tired of reading about basements and showers. All of my suggestions may be starting to sound like commandments: You should do this. You should not do that. You may feel that you do not need more rules and regulations—you live with plenty already. Your boss orders your actions at work, traffic signals rule you on the road, the government tells you how much how much tax you must pay on your purchases. Why should you let me dictate your actions at home?

The answer is this: You should follow these suggestions because they can make you well. I know that they are effective. Every day I see and treat people whose health and comfort are adversely affected by allergic exposures at home. Many took actions that eliminated these exposures. Their stories may help you understand that you too must search out and change these exposures. Let's meet some of my patients and hear their stories.

The Wall Came Tumbling Down

It was a typical day in my office and my next patient was a typical patient, except, perhaps, for his dress and manner. He was a handsome man, with brown sports coat and tan trousers tastefully matched with a light brown shirt and red striped tie. He carried himself well, he spoke carefully and clearly, he approached our interview with humor and confidence.

With his manner and dress, I visualized him living on the eighteenth floor of a very expensive apartment building. I was wrong about where he lived, and where he lived dictated his symptoms.

Dan told me that, no matter the season, his nose was continually congested. The congestion worsened in the spring and fall, seasons when the air is filled with tree, grass, and ragweed pollens. Through the winter his congestion was less severe but persistent. In addition to the congestion, he also suffered from heavy postnasal discharge, often so heavy that he continually coughed to remove this discharge from his throat and upper air passages.

An itchy nose made him sneeze frequently. An itchy face made him scratch often, especially in peculiar areas where the itch was most uncomfortable, his left cheek and the tip of his nose. All these symptoms started years ago when he was living in a basement apartment.

Now, instead of living in the eighteenth-floor apartment that I visualized, Dan is living in another basement. We talked about the problems of living in a basement where the concrete slab of the building forms the floor, how the humidity from the ground rises through the slab to moisten the air and the pad, carpet, and upholstered furniture that rest on the slab. It encourages the growth of dust mites and mold, which then cause the congestion, itchiness, and other symptoms that Dan suffers.

Dan's skin tests agreed with this, showing allergy to dust mites, mold, and pollen. After reading the test, I told him that it would be best for him to leave this basement apartment. How long did he plan to live there? He replied that he did not plan to move in the near future, so we decided to strengthen him against this exposure by using allergy injections. After three months of treatment, he returned to tell me whether the injections were helping him.

Indeed, the injections quieted his symptoms nicely and Dan was pleased with the help they gave him—his itch and cough were both much relieved. However, his improvement was not due only to the injections.

After our first visit Dan returned to his living quarters and examined them closely. He decided that they were as musty as I suspected. When he tried to tell his roommates about this mustiness, they doubted him. This doubt faded when he found convincing evidence of mustiness. One day when he was showering in his basement bathroom, he noticed a loose tile. When he poked at it, it fell right off the wall. He moved to the next tile and then the next tile—they also separated easily from the wall. When he had accumulated a little pile of tiles, he looked at the denuded wall and saw that it was covered with black and white mold growth.

When he showed his roommates the results of his barehanded demolition, they agreed there was a problem. They tore down the shower wall and rebuilt it properly and Dan's congestion and itchiness lessened as the repaired shower decreased his exposure to mites and mold. He feels much better. He plans to move soon from this basement apartment into a new home that he is building.

Dan's story interested me because it carries an important message for every homeowner, especially those affected by allergy. Do not place showers in basements. If you do, watch for conditions that allow the growth of mold. Correct them. Your corrections can significantly slow the growth of the mold that makes you ill.

Sara's Story

Sara's experience was quite similar. She is one of my many patients who suffer from recurrent sinus infections. When I evaluate these patients, I closely question them about their homes and workplaces, looking for a source of mustiness with its attendant mold, yeast, algae, and bacteria. I believe that these microorganisms and their bioaerosols cause my patients' sinus infections. In Sara's case, I wondered if her home had a source of mustiness that kept her infected. A surprising event confirmed this suspicion.

Her daughter, as she was showering, leaned against the shower's soap dish. It fell down. She reported the downed soap dish to her parents, and when they checked the shower, they saw that in the hole where the soap dish had been attached the wall was black with mold.

Sara and her husband tore apart the wall and discovered that the moldiness extended through the moisture-resistant drywall all the way back to the basement foundation wall. They tore out the entire wall and replaced it with concrete backer board, which is the correct base for a shower. They then installed a plastic surround in the shower stall and caulked it to prevent water seepage.

Sara vividly describes the scene when she and her husband carried the moldy tiles and wall material out of the house. The refuse stank with an overwhelming smell of moldiness. As she carried the moldy trash in her bucket she realized it caused the foul odor she had noticed while in the basement. She told me, "Now that the shower is repaired, the whole basement smells much better. When I am in the basement my nose doesn't stuff up and my head doesn't hurt."

Her repeated sinus infections also stopped.

Mikki's Basement

Mikki's story is similar to Dan and Sara's but with one grand improvement. Let's hear her story and then discuss the improvement.

I was treating Mikki for the usual symptoms that my patients bring to me—stuffiness, headaches, and tiredness. In Mikki's case, she suffers nasal congestion and sinus and migraine headaches. She also wheezes. She is a very sensitive person, not only reacting to her allergies but also reacting to our allergy injection treatments—we are forced to use only very low dosage allergy injections in her treatment. When we tried to increase these low doses, she developed angry red swellings at the site of the injections.

In spite of this sensitivity, the injection treatment helped to relieve her symptoms but she still suffered consequences of her allergies, including far too many headaches and far too much tiredness. Then, one day she returned to tell me that she felt much better. Knowing that my treatment could not account for this improvement I asked her, "Tell me what happened, why do you feel better?"

"I'm happy to tell you," she said. "The house that I live in has a basement that was remodeled in about 1970. The previous owners had paneled and insulated the basement walls. Ever since I bought the house, I noticed the basement had a peculiar, although not very strong, smell. I wondered if the smell had anything to do with the chest pain and difficult breathing that affected me whenever I was in the basement."

Mikki and her husband noticed the blistering paint covering the basement walls and wondered about the cause of it. Could water be behind the paneling? They removed some of the paneling and got an unpleasant surprise. Blackish green mold where the paneling faced the wall, coloring the insulation and the basement wall behind it. Horrible! The smell? Equally horrible.

They did what needed to be done—they gutted the basement. They removed the drywall and paneling. They removed the moldy insulation. They removed the studs that were deteriorating with rot. They hauled all of this smelly, moldy material out of the basement.

Now when Mikki is in the basement, she no longer suffers. Appreciating her much improved health, she is pointing all her efforts toward further basement repair. She plans to power wash and seal the walls. She will not reinstall insulation and paneling. She will no longer need to wonder if the wall behind the paneling is leaking, she can just go into the basement, look at the wall, and see any leak. She will no longer have to worry about the condition of the carpeting, as the basement will have no carpeting.

I thoroughly agree with Mikki's plans. Because of her actions, I expect that her stuffiness, wheezing, tiredness, and her sinus and migraine headaches will decrease nicely over the next several years. As I agree with her actions and as I delight in her good health, I also think with sadness about all the suffering people with moldy basements. Their basements probably look beautiful with bright carpet on the floor, upholstered furniture tastefully arranged in various rooms, and attractive paneling and paint on the walls. But woe the mold that lurks behind the beauty.

Rose's Referral

A letter I sent to my patient's referring doctors can perhaps best tell the next patient story. Of all the patients I have told you about, Rose's husband acted most decisively and completely to end a health menace.

Dear Doctors:

I have been treating Rose since 1991. During this time she has lived in residences that caused much of her allergic illnesses. She lived in apartments where she could see mold on the walls; these apartments made her cough and suffer painful headaches. The coughing and headaches were both frequent and debilitating. In 1995 she moved to her present home, and in this home her nasal congestion, headaches, and coughing continued without letup.

One reason for Rose's symptoms was the condition of the basement. Fearing that the basement was moldy, Rose's husband removed paneling and insulation from the walls all the way to the cinder blocks. He found heavy contamination with mold. He noticed water leaking through the cinder block wall, and to stop it he dug a trench around the outside of the house and installed a drainage system and proper backfill. He also broke through the basement floor and installed an interior drainage system. Further, he removed all the basement partition walls and the dropped ceiling. All of these repairs are working and the basement is drier and does not smell moldy. Rose is noticing some relief of her symptoms and this relief should continue to improve over the next several years. Her son, who also suffers allergy symptoms (coughing, stuffy nose, and headaches) is recovering nicely.

That Rose is very sensitive to mold was dramatically demonstrated last summer after a two-hour visit to an underground cave. Following the visit she suffered wheezing, headaches, nasal stuffiness, and a severe cough. These symptoms made her so sick that serious consideration was given to treating her with cortisone. She finally recovered after three months. This prolonged illness after a major mold exposure is typical for the allergic person.

Rose will continue to receive allergy injections. This treatment, plus the lower allergen levels that she will breathe as a result of the extensive home repair, should help her feel far more comfortable.

Sincerely,
William E. Walsh, M.D.

Reflections on Our Stories

I believe that you will agree with me that these stories are dramatic. I chose them for that reason. Although dramatic, they are not unusual. I have hundreds of patients who live above musty basements, and no treatment of mine, although helpful, will end their tiredness, stuffiness, wheezing, and headaches. Correcting the conditions at home that make them suffer will end these symptoms.

Many of my patients discovered moldiness in rotting floors, ceilings, and walls of bathrooms and showers. When they removed the rotten wood their symptoms improved. If you crave the same good health they found, you must search for and repair these conditions if they affect your house.

I do not have as many stories about patients living in homes with moldy walls caused by roof leaks, a subject we will cover next. My stories are few about water let into the walls by wet brick or stucco, as I live in an area with mostly wooden homes. They are also few about the tightly insulated modern homes where unbalanced ventilation sucks in moisture that condenses on and in the walls, spurring mold growth in these walls as it passes through, or are inadequately ventilated, trapping moisture inside the home. These homes exist and I believe many of my patients live in them. My lack of stories arises not from their rarity, but from the difficulty of identifying these houses. How easy it is to miss mold in walls covered with paint and wallpaper. Please be alert and find these conditions if they exist in your home.

So far we have examined the basement and first and second floors of the house and seen how mold and mites can grow and cause allergic sickness. As I mentioned above, now we will pay attention to the walls and roof of the home and briefly review the experience of some of my patients who lived with moldy walls and defective roofs.

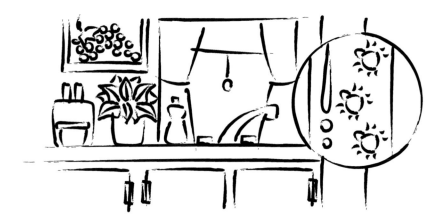

CHAPTER 9

The Roof and Walls of the House

NO ASPECT OF THE HOUSE frustrates an allergist's search for the cause of his patients' illnesses more than a home's walls. You cannot look inside them and many of the allergy-causing problems they harbor hide from the homeowner who cannot then report them to the allergist.

In my practice, this is often the case. Many of my patients suffer symptoms that suggest they live in moldy houses. Yet, my questions about their houses reveal no obvious source of mustiness. Lacking this obvious source of the mustiness, I then suspect that my patients' homes have moldy walls. Unfortunately, because walls can hide their mold under painted or paneled surfaces, I cannot discover if my suspicion is correct. This uncertainty frustrates me and prevents me from suggesting corrections that would help my patients.

Equally as frustrating as the walls is the roof. In this chapter I will try to give you some suggestions about discovering and correcting roof and wall problems.

My Patients' Stories of Wall and Roof Problems

Perhaps I can best help you understand the threat posed by the walls and roof by telling you what some of my patients found when they searched their walls and roofs. In each of the cases I describe, my treatment had failed to relieve their symptoms and I wondered why. My patients discovered the reason.

Jane found that a recently added porch allowed water to penetrate the wall at the porch-house junction. This junction had to be repaired, and the studs and moldy insulation removed and replaced. Once these defects were corrected, her symptoms resolved.

Debra struggled for years with unremitting headaches. While searching for the cause of her illnesses, she found a spot of mold on the wall of a closet. Removing the wall and replacing the insulation finally allowed her headaches to subside.

Cecilia noticed mold on the ceiling and down one wall of her bedroom. Repairing the roof leak that allowed rain and snowmelt to wet the wall, followed by repairing the wall and ceiling and replacing ceiling insulation, finally stopped her wheezing and headaches.

Mary's nose was so blocked by allergic swelling that neither allergy medication nor allergy injections helped her breathe. When she removed the kitchen cabinets in her apartment to install new ones she found behind them a solid sheet of black mold. We suspect that the brick siding of the apartment building became wet when it rained and transferred this moisture into the wall cavity and hence onto the inside wall. She quickly moved from this apartment and over the next several years her blocked nose gradually opened.

In each of these cases hidden mold exposure perpetuated a most uncomfortable allergic illness. If your house has these hidden mold exposures, you should try to discover and correct them.

The Roof

I feel peculiar telling you how to care for your roof because if you ever saw me actually standing on a roof, you would see a white-faced, shaking allergist with his eyes tightly shut. I suffer from such fear of heights that I find a six-foot stepladder five feet too high. However, I should comment about roofs, not because I am an expert in their care and maintenance but because they are so important that they cannot be ignored.

You must have an intact roof over your head to shed rain and snow. Otherwise, water that is allowed to pass into the house will wet and rot the wood studs and insulation in the walls. Water from rain and snow will similarly wet and mold the ceiling materials that the roof should protect. An obvious entry for this water is a roof defect such as a missing shingle or inadequate flashing. Flat roofs are especially susceptible to such defects; you should avoid the home with a flat roof.

A second, less obvious way for water to enter the attic during the winter is through humidity arising from inside the house. It passes into the attic through openings created by chimneys, vent pipes, and interior partitions. Openings are also created by cracks opened in the attic or roof by the deflection of floors and the settling of foundations. In winter, once this moisture enters the attic space, it condenses and freezes on the cold attic surfaces and on warm winter days it melts and flows down the wall spaces and drips onto the attic insulation and the ceiling below, encouraging the growth of mold.

Inspecting the Roof

To keep your attic dry, check the roof several times a year to detect any damaged or missing shingles. Look for other roof damage that disrupts its integrity. If, like me, you cannot stand heights, examine a slanted roof by using a pair of binoculars with your feet firmly planted on the ground.

Examining the roof from the outside is not the only way to determine its integrity. Go into the attic and look at the underside of the roof. If you do not examine this surface, the roof—like the walls—will hide its defects from you. In summer, inspect your attic with a good flashlight during or after a rainstorm and check for any water on the underside of the roof, dripping down trusses, or wetting the insulation. With the light off, you can see if any sunlight leaks through, indicating a hole in the roof. In winter, look for moisture frozen on attic surfaces. If you find water or ice there, correct the defect that allows moisture to enter the attic space. It is true that in many modern homes the attic space is limited and examining it is inconvenient—and uncomfortable. But you must examine it. If you have any problem examining the roof, an examination by a professional roofer is money well spent.

Gutters, Downspouts, and Landscape Drainage

At this time, let's return to directing water away from your house. Intact and well-functioning gutters and downspouts are essential unless you have a perfectly designed and maintained landscape that drains rain and snowmelt away from the house. If gutters, downspouts, or landscape drainage have any defects, they will allow rain and snowmelt to drop beside the house, seep into the ground, and pool under the basement slab. From there, the water then oozes up through the basement floor and/or leaks through the walls unless its movement is blocked by an intact moisture barrier and an adequate drainage system.

Even with intact gutters and downspouts, never assume that the water they discharge will drain away from the house. I did and I was wrong. I wondered why my garage so often smelled like a swamp. Then, during a heavy rain, I happened to be idly looking at the downspout near the garage while it discharged its water into the backyard. Much to my surprise I found that the water from the downspout, instead of draining away, pooled and then sank into the soil under the garage. Diverting the downspout to the side of the garage with good drainage allowed it to run down a hill and away from the house. Now my garage smells dry.

On the other side of my house, poor landscape drainage also allowed water to pool and seep into the basement. I cut a swale through the ground to a downhill slope to drain this area.

Ventilation, Insulation, and Vapor Barriers

To lessen moisture from condensation in the attic, provide adequate ventilation that keeps the attic space dry. Proper roof ventilation not only helps dissipate the moisture that accumulates during the winter, it also cools the attic in hot weather. Continuous ridge and soffit vents with wind-wash barriers that supply even ventilation in the attic are recommended. If you are building a new home, before the drywall is attached, a vapor barrier will be installed on the ceiling below the attic. This vapor barrier plus added insulation makes the ceiling airtight and reduces the movement of warm, moist house air into the attic in winter, inhibits moisture condensation there, and helps prevent ice dams from forming along the eaves of sloped roofs.

Always choose suitable ceiling insulation that will not produce fibers and dust or provide habitat to insects or vermin. The best insulation is fiberglass as it resists the loss of insulation that occurs if attic insulation becomes wet. Raised-heel or energy roof trusses provide more space for insulation and help prevent ice dams and shingle damage by allowing insulation to extend over the top of the sidewall.

One of the greatest sources of attic moisture is the recessed ceiling light. The light fixture acts like a chimney, drawing moist house air into the attic. If you have these lights, remove them or ensure that they are tightly sealed. Build a box over each fixture and add extra insulation around the box to prevent this chimney effect. Alternatively, replace the fixture with an air-tight recessed fixture rated for contact with insulation.

Other bypasses that allow house moisture to escape into the attic include the places where pipes and cables pass through the ceiling into the attic. It's a good idea to seal these with expanding foam insulation.

The Walls

As you can see from my patients' stories, moisture in the walls of the house that encourages mold growth is a disaster. This moisture can come from an excessively humid house where the humidity in the air penetrates the walls and in winter freezes in the wall cavities. It can come from the rain and snowmelt admitted by a defective roof. It can infiltrate the wall space from a defective junction between a new addition and the house. Wet brick, especially in older buildings without proper vapor barriers, may transfer moisture into the wall cavity behind the brick. Thus, the possible sources of wetness are many.

Sometimes you can discover this moisture by examining the outside of the house. If you find areas of peeling paint on the walls, suspect that moisture is entering the walls behind the area of peeling.

Several sources caused wall wetness and mold in my house and distressed me greatly. I noticed a swamp-like smell in the walls of a bedroom and couldn't imagine where it came from. Much to my surprise, one winter when I was in the attic I found snow on the insulation at the top of that wall. How did the snow fall onto the insulation? It blew into the attic through a vent placed on the attic wall. The snow dropped onto the insulation and, on warm days, melted and seeped into the wall cavity, spurring the growth of mold and algae. When we replaced the insulation and permanently closed the vent, the smell disappeared. I also added extra vents in the roof soffit and a continuous ridge vent to more adequately vent the attic.

Then I noticed an area on the wall and ceiling in a closet on my porch crumbling from water dripping from above. It took me several months to find the source of that water. It came from a missing triangle of wood that should have been replaced in the siding of the house where it met the roof of the porch. When rain blew onto the wall from the east, the water ran through the hole into the wall and dripped on the porch closet ceiling. To the best of my knowledge, this piece had been missing for years. I replaced the wood and the crumbling stopped.

The last source of wall moisture in my house was a poorly fitted window that allowed water to enter the wall it was mounted in.

I hope that these examples show you that, even if you see no obvious source, you can never be sure that the stuffiness, headaches, or other miseries that you suffer do not arise from your home. If you suffer these symptoms, the walls of your home may not be your friends.

Windows and Doors That Resist Condensation

The windows and doors of a house should resist the movement of cold air into the home. This heat-conserving ability is called the U-factor. The windows should have a U-factor of .35 in a cold-climate home. Features to look for in an energy-efficient window include low-e insulation; a sealed, gas-filled space between panes; and warm-edge spacers between the panes to minimize the transfer of heat and cold. *Note:* A new measure of window efficiency is the Solar Heat Gain Coefficient, which measures the efficiency of the window at preventing heat transmission into the home. This is particularly useful for southern, plains, and western homes.

The installer should seal the windows and doors to the air-infiltration barrier to protect the continuity of this barrier. Any break in continuity leaves a space where moisture-laden air may be sucked into your house if fans and combustion appliances are not properly balanced and create negative pressure. The air sucked into your house to relieve this negative pressure may deposit its moisture in the wall cavities or around the windows as condensate, wetting and molding the wall or window. In addition, the windows and doors should be properly flashed to direct rain and snowmelt away and keep it from penetrating the wall. Inside, the vapor barrier should be securely fastened to the window and door jambs to prevent moist indoor air from migrating into the wall cavities.

Reflections

We looked at the walls and roof of a house and saw how, for the allergic person, they can make a home suitable or unsuitable. Through my patients' experiences you have seen that these defects in their homes truly cause distressing allergic illnesses. You have also seen how these defects can be so frustratingly difficult to detect. Often a qualified home inspector (ASHI-certified) can help you find defects that need to be corrected. An inspector's services can be well worth the fee you will pay.

From this information I hope that you have learned that if you suffer allergic illness and can find no cause, suspect that mustiness hides in the attic or walls. Once you suspect this mustiness, search for it. May your search be successful.

Next let's turn our attention to what the addition of a pet to a home can do to the health of its occupants.

What You Want in Walls and Roofs

Feature	Look for...	Avoid...
Roof and attic	...a roof that is in good condition and free of leaks. ...adequate soffit and ridge vents. ...adequate and properly placed insulation. ...all bypasses from the house into the attic have been sealed.	...a leaky and/or unventilated roof. ...inadequate attic insulation. ...unsealed bypasses that allow moisture to escape from the house into the attic.
Gutters and downspouts	...well-maintained, properly sized and installed gutters that truly drain water from the roof away from the house.	...a house without gutters.
Walls	...intact siding and properly flashed doors and windows.	...a house where improper construction techniques allow water to pass into the walls, creating moisture problems that will make you sick.
Windows and doors	...energy-efficient windows and doors. ...proper installation, including flashing and sealing to the air-infiltration barrier and vapor barrier.	...leaky, uninsulated windows. ...unflashed windows and doors that allow rain and snowmelt to penetrate the walls of the house.

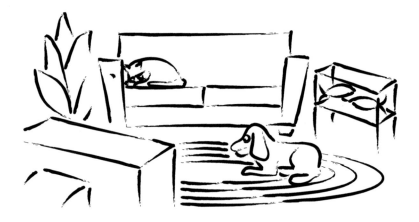

CHAPTER 10

Pets in the Home

I MADE ONE OF THE BIGGEST MISTAKES of my practice early in my years as an allergist. Fresh from my training in the excellent allergy fellowship program at the Mayo Clinic, I felt that I knew allergy well. I saw my field in black and white, with no gray areas. For example, I saw clearly that no animals should be in the home of the allergy sufferer. Pompously I told patients, "I will not treat you if you keep your dog or cat."

Much to my delight, my patients returned to tell me that they had eliminated pets from their homes. How proud I was to bring such an obviously correct improvement to my patients' homes!

Then, one of my patients gave my certainty a grievous blow and I started seeing shades of gray. She told me that, after several years of treatment, she was feeling fine in spite of keeping her pet. She admitted that she had lied to me about eliminating the animal so that I would treat her with allergy injections.

This experience taught me much. First, people often will not give up a pet, even if the pet causes allergic symptoms. Second, I can successfully treat patients who live with pets even if they are allergic to these pets. Last but not least, I should never force patients into feeling they have to lie to me, as it damages the trust so necessary in the doctor-patient relationship.

Now I advise patients to remove pets from the home, but I do not require them to do so. I do not even expect them to eliminate pets, as most will not. My thoughts are shared by many allergists as shown by Stanley Coren of the Department of Psychology at the University of British Columbia in Vancouver, Canada. In a study of 341 adults, he found that only about 25 percent of patients advised to eliminate pets from the home did so; about 75 percent kept them. Even more striking was a study of 122 patients treated for prolonged periods. Of those patients allergic to pets whose animals had died during treatment, 86 (70 percent) had replaced the animal with a new dog or cat.

The only patients that I try hard to separate from their pets are those who suffer from asthma. Much research indicates that exposure to pets in pet-sensitive asthmatics increases the inflammatory condition of the lungs and makes the patients more sensitive to other allergic and infectious exposures. As asthma can be a life-threatening illness, any action that reduces its ability to sicken a patient should be pursued with vigor. Moreover, asthma is more common in the children of parents with asthma and evidence suggests that pet exposure in the home increases the chances that the children will develop asthma. Eliminating the pet in families with asthmatic parents may prevent this asthma.

With these thoughts in mind, let's examine pet allergy in more detail and look at methods to lessen its impact.

Where Dog and Cat Allergy Comes From
Although we think of animal allergy as involving a pet's hair, this is really a minor source of allergy. Although the hair or fur can collect

pollen, dust, mold, and other allergens and bring them into the home, it is not the major source of animal allergen.

The major source of animal allergen is proteins that the pet produces to make its own muscles, blood cells, enzymes, and all the other body components that keep it alive. We humans also produce proteins to make our own body components, but our proteins are slightly different from our pets'. Our immune system accepts the proteins we make and does not attack them (except in autoimmune illnesses). However, it will attack proteins that we do not make, causing allergic illness.

We encounter these pet proteins when we breathe the airborne particles of saliva, dander (dead skin flakes), urine, and feces of an animal. The proteins gain entrance to the urine and feces by leaking from the pet's body into the urine and feces through the urinary system walls or the walls of the intestinal tract. Cells shed from these walls also add to the allergy proteins of the urine and feces. All breeds of animals shed these proteins—there are no "hypoallergenic" breeds of cats or dogs.

The proteins from pet urine, feces, dander, and saliva eventually dry out and then float in the air and land on the lining of the eyes or nose; breathing them draws them into the lungs. Although most people react only if the animal is present in the room, others with more severe sensitivity suffer these symptoms from animal allergens carried on the clothes of pet owners.

Symptoms include sneezing, wheezing, tearing, nasal discharge, and itching of the nose, eyes, and throat. Touching an animal may make the skin itch and raise a swollen, red rash (hives). These symptoms can appear quickly, sometimes within minutes of exposure, or they may start slowly and become severe eight to twelve hours later.

Reducing Your Exposure to Dog and Cat Allergens

If you are allergic to your pet, and you decide to keep it, you will find it difficult to avoid its allergy-causing proteins. The difficulty arises because animals are not clean. To understand this, visualize your child acting like a dog or cat.

Instead of a daily bath, your child does not bathe for weeks. To substitute for the bathing, he licks himself industriously several times a day and does not wash off the areas he licks. Instead of using the toilet, he urinates and defecates into a box in your home or on the lawn or in a kennel outside. He never cleans himself after relieving himself so particles of fecal matter can cling to his hair. Further, it concerns him not at all that he steps in his droppings as he plays and he never cleans his feet when he reenters the home.

You would have a long and serious talk with this child and change his ways quickly. You do not tolerate unclean children. With a pet, you have to tolerate it.

With these rather icky thoughts in mind, let's review favorable and unfavorable actions you can take to reduce dog or cat allergy. I have arranged these actions with the most effective listed first and less effective actions listed further down the list. Finally, detrimental actions end the list. Please understand that I appreciate your love of your pet and regret that you must consider these actions.

- Find another home for your pet.

- If you keep a pet, follow meticulous environmental control measures, especially in the bedroom, to lower your exposure to mite, mold, and food allergies. (See below, bucket of allergy.)

- Avoid close contact with the pet. Restricting the pet to the yard and not allowing it in the home is less effective than not having a pet. If you restrict it to the yard, levels of pet allergen will be lower in your home, but your home will have some level of animal allergen because you will carry it indoors on your clothes.

- Restrict the pet to the unfinished basement.

- Restrict the pet to the basement and uncarpeted kitchen.

- Allow the pet to be in the uncarpeted first floor of your two-story house.

- Remove all carpeting from the house and allow the pet to roam the house while excluding it from the bedroom.

- Allow the cat or dog free entrance to selected carpeted areas of the home while excluding it from your bedroom.

- Allow the pet free run of a carpeted home, including your bedroom.

- Play with and pet the animal, allowing it to climb on furniture and to rest on your lap.

Carpeting with Pets

I place emphasis on carpets because they are a reservoir of cat and dog saliva, dander, urine, and fecal material. The allergenic proteins from these sources work deeply into the carpet and any associated padding and cannot be removed by vacuuming as vacuuming does not clean the protein that has migrated into these lower levels. In fact, vacuuming can stir up small allergen particles, which can move through the vacuum bag into the air.

In the carpet, cat and dog allergenic proteins join the proteins emanating from dust mites, mold, algae, and yeast. Together, they exude a witch's brew of allergic proteins that gain entry to the air you breathe, increasing the ability of dog and cat proteins to bring you distressing symptoms.

If you are animal sensitive and move into a home that housed animals, remove and dispose of all the carpeting and any upholstered furniture left behind as they were probably contaminated by their presence. It can take weeks or months of cleaning to lower the amount of animal allergens in fabrics and carpets; these allergens may persist for a year or more after the animal has been removed.

The Bucket of Allergy

This brings up the concept of the *bucket of allergy*. In this concept, you carry a bucket to hold all the allergic exposures that might set off your allergic symptoms. If your allergic exposures are few, they easily fit into this bucket and you suffer no symptoms. Only when your exposures are too many to fit into your bucket will you sneeze, wheeze, or suffer headaches. It is to your advantage to keep the bucket as empty as you can.

Perhaps, if you are not exposed much to allergenic dust mites, mold, yeast, algae, and foods, your bucket will have lots of room for your pet exposure. You can tolerate your animal without symptoms. Therefore, if you keep your pet, try as hard as you can to remove other allergic exposures and avoid foods that aggravate your allergic symptoms.

You can take other actions to minimize your exposure to the allergenic proteins of your dog or cat, but the effectiveness of the following measures is uncertain.

- Wash the dog or cat once or twice a week. If you plan to wash your pet regularly, consult with your veterinarian regarding care of the animal's skin to prevent excessive dryness. Also, have a non-allergic family member brush the pet outside to remove loose hair and allergens.

- Purchase a pet such as a turtle, hermit crab, fish, snake, or other animal without fur or feathers. A note of caution: Many of these pets must be kept in a moist, moldy environment such as an aquarium and this mold will contribute to the mold level of the home's air. At the very least, keep them out of the bedroom. In the case of aquariums, if they have an aerating device, the air escaping from the aquarium into the home air will be humid and may contain high levels of algae, yeast, mold, and bacteria. Aquariums with aerators should not be in the home of an allergy sufferer. A small fish bowl without an aerator may be acceptable.

Rabbits, Mice, Rats, Hamsters, Guinea Pigs, and Birds

Allergies to mice, rats, hamsters, and guinea pigs are common and these animals should not be in the home of an allergic person. If they are, keep them out of the bedroom and ask a non-allergic family member to clean the cage as their droppings are a potent source of the allergenic protein that causes allergy to animals.

Similarly, bird's allergens are found in their feces and urine; these droppings can also be a source of bacteria, dust, and mold. Dropped to the bottom of the cage, the urine and feces dry there. The movements of the bird then blow the dried droppings from the cage into the home. It also blows the bird's dander and saliva through the home. Birds should not be in the home of the allergic person. If they are, clean the cage before the droppings dry.

A Note of Reassurance

Although a pet in the home of the allergic person is inadvisable, practical experience shows that many homes contain them. As I mentioned above, not only do they contain them, few pet owners will eliminate them. If the pet owner's sensitivity to the animals is minor, as is often the case, the pet owner can tolerate the exposure. Following the above suggestions can help sustain this tolerance. Only in the case of the asthmatic sensitive to animals, or in the case of the severely sensitive person, does the elimination spell the difference between health and illness.

Somewhat confusing the issue is research that indicates that children born into homes with cats, and with high exposure to these cats, often show a state of tolerance to cats. They also are less likely to develop asthma. This observed lower risk of wheezing among exposed children is only observed in children exposed to cats very early in life, at birth and soon after, and suggests this early exposure has a protective effect in this age group. Exposure to pets in older children appears to slightly increase their risk of asthma and wheezing.

A possible reason for a decreased possibility of asthma in the very young is that children exposed to increased levels of germs in very early life may be more resistant to developing asthma. Close exposure to germs carried by cats may induce this resistance.

These studies showing a tolerance to cats in the very young may be in error—some design flaws in the studies may have led to error in the results. For instance, this result may have arisen because parents most likely to have a child with asthma do not keep cats; those less likely to have a child with asthma keep them. Also, we do not know if this possible tolerance may be broken by a period without cats and, on reintroduction, the resulting cat sensitivity then may lead to pronounced symptoms.

The above thoughts do not mean that you can keep a cat without suffering symptoms if you are cat sensitive. You will suffer if you keep it. The only question is how much you will suffer. Nor does it mean that a cat will not speed the appearance of asthma in a child exposed to it. We cannot predict which children will be more stimulated to wheeze and which children will be more resistant.

With these thoughts in mind, we can give this reassurance to some pet owners: In many cases, allergic people can live comfortably with animals.

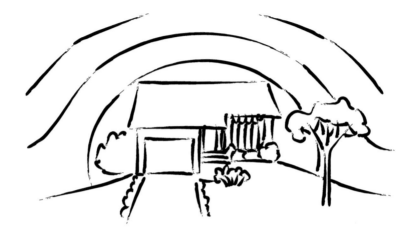

CHAPTER 11

The "Perfect" Home
for the Allergic Person

AS WE DISCUSSED IN PREVIOUS CHAPTERS, your home can generate airborne allergen exposures, bioaerosols, that are nasty. How do you prevent these exposures, and what is the perfect home for you? Perhaps there is no "perfect" home. No matter how hard you try to make it perfect, mistakes in location or construction may prevent perfection. Defects that arise as the house ages may also counteract your efforts. However, you should not stop either trying to build this home, trying to discover a home that possesses the virtues you seek, or repairing the home where you now live.

In this, our last chapter, I will depart from the lists of commands that so far fill this book. No more Thou shalt do this and Thou shalt not do that. Instead, I will describe some aspects of the home where you should live. While I review many of the subjects we covered earlier, I will build this home in your mind, step-by-step.

- Your home site is open and landscape drainage is good. It is distant from woods and water.

- Testing shows the water table to be at least one foot below the basement slab.

- In new construction you have installed an adequate vapor barrier over the ground before the slab is poured. You placed a good moisture barrier and insulation over the outside of the foundation walls. A footing drain is in place—and a sump pump if necessary—to carry away water that would otherwise enter the basement.

- If you are building a new home, you seal the walls of the house with a vapor barrier. The sealing includes all areas where moisture can enter or exit the house, including where walls meet and the floor of the attic. Installing an air exchanger in this new home avoids the need to perforate the roof to install bathroom vent fans. A kitchen exhaust fan is installed to remove grease and other cooking by-products.

- The basement is open, without partition walls and a decorative ceiling covering the trusses or joists that support the floor above the basement. The floor is covered with ceramic tile or painted with a sealer that retards humidity passing through the slab. A sealer is also applied to the walls and no insulation, studs, or drywall cover the basement walls. You can easily see any water leaking from the walls or seeping up from the floor; you can mop up the water and repair the condition that caused the leak. In new home construction, if you finished the basement, you employed a painstaking and knowledgeable craftsman and you pray the basement never floods.

- You have installed a sealed-combustion forced-air furnace and water heater. The air cleaner is efficient and you connected a heat-conserving air exchanger to the ductwork. The air exchanger is carefully calibrated to supply replacement air to replace the air drawn from the house by any vented appliance. An air conditioner provides refuge from the summer's humidity and pollen. You sealed the ductwork, and it adequately vents the entire house, including the basement and large closets, with supply and return ducts in every room.

- The home has a carefully balanced supply of makeup air to allow the various exhaust fans to work properly and safely.

- In the basement you placed a washer, a dryer vented to the outside, and a workbench. The dehumidifier operates there from spring to late fall. Any furniture is plastic or wood, not upholstered, and you store moldable material in plastic containers. You placed no carpets in the basement, if present they are throw or area rugs that you properly maintain.

- If you must keep a pet indoors, you restrict its access to the house. No pet-protein-catching carpeting is in the house. You also will not have carpeting if your allergic symptoms are severe, such as persistent asthma. If your allergies are mild and you do not keep pets, newer, well-maintained carpets are acceptable as long as they do not rest on a concrete slab in contact with the ground. You use a central vacuum system that vents outside or a vacuum with a HEPA filter or double or triple-layered bag. You do not steam-clean the carpet.

- You cook with an electric stove. A fireplace, if present, is tightly sealed to prevent downdrafts or escape of fumes or gas into the home.

- Your bedroom is on the second floor, contains no carpeting, and your mattress, box springs, and pillow are covered with dust-proof encasings. You wash the bedding materials weekly in hot water. A free-standing HEPA air filter operates in your bedroom while you sleep.

- The roof is intact, and gutters and downspouts carry water away from the house. If they are absent, you carefully design and maintain your landscaping to carry water away from the house. The walls are intact, dry, and free of mold.

May Your House Shelter You and Help Keep You Healthy

After years of treating patients whose homes make them sick, I so wanted to tell you how you can avoid this same sickness. I have treated many patients whose debilitating migraine headaches, asthma, chronic sinus infections, and other illness began or worsened after moving to a musty home. I have also shared the triumph and happiness of patients who corrected the home defects that make them sick or moved to a healthy home. I wish you the triumph and happiness of living in a home suited for you.

You may not have the opportunity to build the "perfect" home or the financial resources to completely repair an older home. However, let me assure you that every step you take to correct your present home will be one more step toward the good health that you deserve. Each step, no matter how small, will be more valuable for your health and well-being than all the expensive medicine lining the pharmacy shelves. Start these steps today; you will be glad that you did.

Bibliography

Apelberg, Benjamin J.; Y. Aoki; and J. J. K. Jaakkola. "Systematic Review: Exposure to Pets and Risk of Asthma and Asthma-Like Symptoms." *Journal of Allergy and Clinical Immunology* 107, no. 3 (2001): 455–60.

Arlian L.G.; J. S. Neal; and D. L. Vyszenski-Moher. "Reducing Relative Humidity to Control the House Dust Mite *Dermatophagoides farinae.*" *Journal of Allergy and Clinical Immunology* 104, no 4 (1999): 852–56.

Arlian, L. G.; J. S. Neal; M. S. Morgan; D. L. Vyszenski-Moher; and T. A. E. Platts-Mills. "The Biology of Dust Mites and the Remediation of Mite Allergens in Allergic Disease." *Journal of Allergy and Clinical Immunology* 107, no.3 (2001): S406–13.

Bush, R. K.; and J. M. Portnoy. "The Role and Abatement of Fungal Allergens in Allergic Diseases." *Journal of Allergy and Clinical Immunology* 107, no. 3 (2001): S430–40.

Chapman, M. D.; and R. A. Wood. "The Role and Remediation of Animal Allergens in Allergic Diseases." *Journal of Allergy and Clinical Immunology* 107, no. 3 (2001): S414–21.

Cooper, J.A. "Environmental Impact of Residential Wood Combustion Emissions and Its Implications." *Journal of the Air Pollution Control Association* 30 (1980): 855–61.

Coren, S. "Allergic Patients Do Not Comply with Doctors' Advice to Stop Owning Pets." [Letter] *British Medical Journal* 314, no. 7079 (1997): 517.

Custovic, A.; B. M. Simpson; A. Simpson; C. Hallam; M. Craven; M. Brutsche; and A. Woodcock. "Manchester Asthma and Allergy Study: Low-Allergen Environment Can Be Achieved and Maintained During Pregnancy and in Early Life." *The Journal of Allergy and Clinical Immunology* 105, no. 2 (2000): 252–58.

Eggleston, P. A.; and L. K. Arruda. "Ecology and Elimination of Cockroaches and Allergens in the Home." *The Journal of Allergy and Clinical Immunology* 107, no. 3 (2001): 422–29.

Eggleston, P. A.; and R. K. Bush, MD. "Environmental Allergen Avoidance: An Overview." *The Journal of Allergy and Clinical Immunology* 107, no. 3 (2001): S403–5.

Hodson, T.; A. Custovic; A. Simpson; M. Chapman; A. Woodcock; and R. Green. "Washing the Dog Reduces Dog Allergen Levels, but the Dog Needs to be Washed Twice a Week." *Journal of Allergy and Clinical Immunology* 103, no. 4 (1999): 581–85

Huss, R. W.; K. Huss; E. N. Squire Jr.; G. B. Carpenter; L. J. Smith; K. Salata; and J. Hershey. "Mite Allergen Control with Acaricide Fails." *The Journal of Allergy and Clinical Immunology* 94, no. 1 (1994): 27–32.

Htut, T.; T. W. Higenbottam; G. W. Gill; R. Darwin; P. B. Anderson; and N. Syed, "Eradication of House Dust Mite from Homes of Atopic Asthmatic Subjects: A Double-Blind Trial." *The Journal of Allergy and Clinical Immunology* 107, no. 1 (2001): 55–60

Jones, A. P. "Asthma and the Home Environment." *Journal of Asthma* 37, no.2 (2000): 103–124.

Kilpeläinena, M.; E. O. Terhoa; H. Heleniusb; and M. Koskenvuoc "Home Dampness, Current Allergic Diseases, and Respiratory Infections Among Young Adults." *Thorax* 56 (2001); 462–67.

Labs, K.; J. Carmody; R. Sterling; L. Shen; Y. J. Huang; and D. Parker. *Building Foundation Design Handbook*. Minneapolis, MN: University of Minnesota, 1988.

Lindfors, A.; M. van Hage-Hamsten; H. Rietz; M. Wickman; and S. L. Nordvall. "Influence of Interaction of Environmental Risk Factors and Sensitization in Young Asthmatic Children." *Journal of Allergy and Clinical Immunology* 104, no. 4 (1999): 755–62.

Lstiburek, J.; and J. Carmody. *Moisture Control Handbook*. New York: Van Nostrand Reinhold Company, 1993.

Platts-Mills, T. A. E.; J. W. Vaughan; M. C. Carter; and J. A. Woodfolk. "The Role of Intervention in Established Allergy: Avoidance of Indoor Allergens in the Treatment of Chronic Allergic Disease." *Journal of Allergy and Clinical Immunology* 106, no. 5 (2000): 787–804.

Platts-Mills, T. A. E.; J. Vaughan; S. Squillace; J. Woodfolk; and R. Sporik. "Sensitisation, Asthma, and a Modified Th2 Response in Children Exposed to Cat Allergen: A Population-Based Cross-Sectional Study." *Lancet* 2001, no. 9258 (2001): 752–56.

Rapp C. M.; and A. K. Alexander. "Reducing Relative Humidity Is a Practical Way to Control Dust Mites and Their Allergens in Homes in Temperate Climates." *The Journal of Allergy and Clinical Immunology* 107, no. 1 (2001): 99–104.

Reed, C. E.; and D. K. Milton. "Endotoxin-Stimulated Innate Immunity: A Contributing Factor for Asthma." *The Journal of Allergy and Clinical Immunology* 108, no. 2 (2001): 157–66.

Tiberg, E.; S. Dreborg; and B. Björkstén. "Allergy to Green Algae (Chlorella) Among Children." *Journal of Allergy and Clinical Immunology* 96, no.2 (1995): 257–59.

Tovey, E. R.; and A. J. Woolcock. "Direct Exposure of Carpets to Sunlight Can Kill All Mites." *Journal of Allergy and Clinical Immunology* 93, no. 6 (1994): 1072–74.

Tovey, E. R.; and G. Marks. "Methods and Effectiveness of Environmental Control." *Journal of Allergy and Clinical Immunology* 103, no. 2 (1999): 179–91.

United States Environmental Protection Agency and the United States Consumer Product Safety Commission Office of Radiation and Indoor Air. "The Inside Story: A Guide to Indoor Air Quality." EPA Document #402-K-93-007, April 1995.

Vaughan, J. W.; J. A. Woodfolk; and T. A. E. Platts-Mills. "Assessment of Vacuum Cleaners and Vacuum Cleaner Bags Recommended for Allergic Subjects." *Journal of Allergy and Clinical Immunology* 104, no. 5 (1999): 1079–83.

Vaughan, J. W.; T. E. McLaughlin; M. S. Perzanowski; and T. A. E. Platts-Mills. "Evaluation of Materials Used for Bedding Encasement: Effect of Pore Size in Blocking Cat and Dust Mite Allergen." *Journal of Allergy and Clinical Immunology* 103, no. 2 (1999) 227–31

Warner, J. A.; J. M. Frederick; T. N. Bryant; C. Weich; G. J. Raw; C. Hunter; F. R. Stephen; D. A. McIntyre; and J. O. Warner. "Mechanical Ventilation and High-Efficiency Vacuum Cleaning: A Combined Strategy of Mite and Mite Allergen Reduction in the

Control of Mite-Sensitive Asthma." *Journal of Allergy and Clinical Immunology* 105, no. 1 (2000): 75–82.

Wood, R. A.; E. F. Johnson; M. L. Van Natta; P. H. Chen; and P. A. Eggleston. "A Placebo-Controlled Trial of a HEPA Air Cleaner in the Treatment of Cat Allergy." *American Journal of Respiratory & Critical Care Medicine.* 158 no. 1 (1998): 115–20.

Woodfolk, J. A.; M. L. Hayden; N. Couture; and T. A. E. Platts-Mills. "Chemical Treatment of Carpets to Reduce Allergen: Comparison of the Effects of Tannic Acid and Other Treatments on Proteins Derived from Dust Mites and Cats." *Journal of Allergy and Clinical Immunology* 96, no. 3 (1995): 325–33.

Additional Resources

MANY OF THE FOLLOWING RESOURCES were invaluable to me while writing this book. Others I discovered while compiling this resource listing. Some of these additional sites contain thoughts and approaches that may differ from those advocated in this book. While I do not necessarily agree with all the content on these sites, I have included them here to offer you different thoughts and approaches to creating a healthy home environment.

Some of the sites in this listing are commercial sites and promote products that the organizations sponsoring the sites wish you to buy. Inclusion of these sites in this list does not imply my endorsement of the products offered for sale. It is my hope that you will apply your own evaluation skills and the guidelines I've laid out in the book to determine if the products offered meet your needs and are a worthwhile purchase that will contribute to making your home healthy.

Professional Organizations

- American Academy of Allergy, Asthma and Immunology
611 East Wells St.,
Milwaukee, WI 53220
website: www.aaaai.org

- American College of Allergy, Asthma & Immunology
85 W. Algonquin Road, Suite 550
Arlington Heights, Illinois 60005
phone: 800-842-7777
public website: www.allergy.mcg.edu
health website: www.medem.com

Indoor Air Quality

- The American Lung Association of Minnesota (ALA) introduced the Health House® concept in 1993 to help individuals learn what they could do in their homes to improve their living environment. To build a Health House®, the association brought together architects, builders, environmental health professionals, indoor air quality specialists, and product manufacturers to design and build a state-of-the-art house that integrates design, construction techniques, and mechanical systems that create a healthier, more energy- and resource-efficient environment. To learn more about their results contact:

  Health House
  490 Concordia Avenue
  St. Paul, MN 55103-2441
  (651) 227-8014
  National Toll Free (877) 521-1491
  Minnesota Toll Free (800) 642-5864
  Fax (651) 281-0242
  E-mail: info@healthhouse.org
  www.healthhouse.org

- Shelter Supply sells building products and technology for building healthier, more energy-efficient homes, including ventilation, waterproofing, and insulation products.

  (800) 762-8399
  www.sheltersupply.com

- Consumer workshops on building a new home may be available through utilities and builders' associations in your state. Call your local utility or builders' association and ask if classes are available.

- Your state may have a department of public service, energy information center. Contact it for publications on building a home.

- The Environmental Protection Agency has many documents concerning indoor air quality available.
  United States Environmental Protection Agency
  1200 Pennsylvania Avenue (1105A)
  Washington, DC 20460
  (202) 564-7333
  Fax (202) 501-1818
  www.epa.gov/iaq/index.html

- Energy Efficiency and Renewable Energy Clearinghouse (EREC)
  P.O. Box 3048 Merrifield, VA 22116
  Voice (USA only): 800-DOE-EREC (363-3732)
  www.eren.doe.gov/consumerinfo/iaq.html

- More information about air cleaners is available from:
  IAQ INFO Clearinghouse
  PO Box 37133
  Washington D.C. 20013-7133
  (703) 356-4020 or 800-438-4318
  fax: (703) 356-5386
  E-mail: iaqinfo@aol.com
  www.epa.gov/iaq/pubs/airclean.html

- Further information on basements can be found at:
  www.extension.umn.edu/distribution/housingandclothing/
      DK7051.html
  www.concretenetwork.com/concrete/basements/
  www.eren.doe.gov/consumerinfo/refbriefs/eb7.html

- For further information on moisture in houses:
  National Research Council Canada
  www.nrc.ca/irc/cbd/cbd231e.html

Green Building

Information about green building, that is, building with an environmental focus, can be found online at the following sites:

- Center for Resourceful Building Technology
  www.crbt.org

- U. S. Green Building Council
  www.usgbc.org

- Environmental Building News
  www.buildinggreen.com

- OIKOS
  www.oikos.com

Allergy-Free Bedrooms

- National Institute of Allergy and Infectious Diseases, National Institutes of Health
  www.niaid.nih.gov/factsheets/dustfree.htm

- Many of the mattress covers, bedclothes, etc. that I discuss can be found in local stores and online.

Cleaning and Cleaning Products

- The Soap and Detergent Association
  www.sdahq.org/health/allergies/

- www.allallergy.net/products/

- www.allergybuyersclub.com

Index

Property of
DeVry University
630 U.S. Highway One
North Brunswick, NJ 08902

RECEIVED JUN 1 4 2006

Also by William E. Walsh, M.D.

Food Allergies: The Complete Guide to Understanding and Relieving Your Food Allergies.

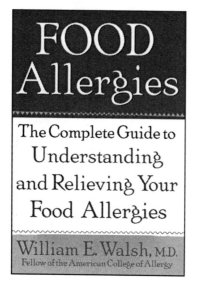

Your home is not the only cause of your allergic pain and discomfort. The foods that you eat can also make you suffer; you can learn to identify these foods and remove them from your diet. In *Food Allergies* Dr. Walsh shares his extensive knowledge of the cause of food allergies, which foods and chemicals to avoid, and which foods will help you feel your best. He shows you how to help yourself. (Published by John Wiley & Sons, Inc. ISBN 0-471-38268-X)

DATE DUE